The Complete Fatfield Diet and Recipe Book

The Complete
FATFIELD
Diet and Recipe Book
EAT MORE – WEIGH LESS

Sally Ann Voak

BCA
LONDON · NEW YORK · SYDNEY · TORONTO

This edition published 1992 by BCA
by arrangement with MICHAEL O'MARA BOOKS

The Complete Fatfield Diet and Recipe Book copyright © 1992 by
Sally Ann Voak

CN 5118

Designed by Mick Keates
Edited by Georgina Evans and Fiona Holman

Typeset by Florencetype Ltd, Kewstoke, Avon
Printed in England by Clays Ltd, St Ives plc

DEDICATION

To Toni, my terrific assistant and the best slimming counsellor
I have ever worked with.

ACKNOWLEDGMENTS

A big thank you to Nerys Hughes, the Presenter of BBC's
'Bazaar'; Erica Griffiths, the Producer; Andy Smith, the
Director; and Val Hudson, the Series Consultant. I'd also like
to thank Susan Collins, the exercise class organiser, Glynis
McGuinness, our home economist who checked my calcula-
tions so patiently, and lastly but most importantly, the villagers
of Fatfield, Tyne and Wear, England. Thank you all for making
the Fatfield Experiment possible – and such fun too!

CONTENTS

FOREWORD

by Dr Gaston L.S. Pawan, D.Sc. (Lond.), FRCPath.
Consultant in Human metabolism and Nutrition

Most overweight fat people would dearly love to be slim, not only because it is fashionable, but because it is well known that overweight increases the risk of heart disease, diabetes, arthritis and many other medical conditions. Physically and psychologically fat people are at a disadvantage. Their mobility, stamina and social life may be affected, and the problems they encounter in our figure- and fashion-conscious society can be formidable.

The question often asked is 'Why does a fat person become fat?' The usual answer given is 'He/she eats too much', and the solution to the problem is therefore 'Eat less and take more exercise' – hence the enormous number of 'slimming diets', exercise programmes and slimming gadgets available on the market. Yet, despite all these aids to slimming, success in losing weight satisfactorily and maintaining a normal bodyweight subsequently, is rare. It is a fact that many fat people may conscientiously follow a calorie-restricted diet for many weeks, often at great personal sacrifice, with some loss of bodyweight, but then on coming off the diet for various reasons, regain the lost weight. A most depressing experience!

Sally Ann Voak, the well-known journalist, author and broadcaster on health and beauty topics, has produced a completely new approach to the slimming problem. Her wide experience of slimmers, their problems and their diets, has led her to reject the usual approach to weight reduction based on the use of smaller meals to reduce calorie intake. Instead, she advocates the consumption of big, hearty, family-sized meals made up of wholesome healthy foods. She argues that in slimming, food should be fun. She shows how large, yet well-balanced, satisfying, calorie-controlled meals can produce steady and enjoyable weight loss. She explains how to relax, be motivated and, if necessary, be one's own counsellor. Simple exercises that are a pleasure to perform are described, and meal plans and recipes suitable for a variety of people, including vegetarians, are given.

I greatly enjoyed reading this book and enthusiastically recommend it. The sensible advice given by Sally Ann Voak should enable the overweight but otherwise healthy person slim successfully, achieve a normal bodyweight, and most importantly, avoid the weight regain so often experienced by slimmers.

Dr Gaston Pawan is Hon. Senior Lecturer, formerly Senior Lecturer, in Metabolism, Department of Medicine, The Middlesex Hospital and Medical School, London. He is Past Chairman of the Association for the Study of Obesity, and Past Chairman of the Board of Studies in Nutrition and Food Science, University of London.

PART ONE

THE DIET

CHAPTER ONE

HOW BIG EATERS
CAN BE BIG LOSERS

Why did you buy this book? Is it because you have tried many, many times to lose weight – and failed? Or is it because the idea of eating *more* and weighing *less* is intriguing?

Maybe, like almost 90 per cent of the population, you are still searching for a diet plan which will help you to slim down for good – a diet that will trim away the inches and the pounds without making you feel fed up, deprived and short-tempered, and one that will also re-train your eating habits so you no longer crave the greasy junk food, alcoholic drinks and sweet snacks that made you put on weight in the first place. The good news is that you have found it!

How can I be so sure? Because, in twenty years of writing, researching and broadcasting about slimming, I have *never* come across a diet that works as brilliantly as the Fatfield Diet does. It is simple, delicious, easy-to-follow and incredibly filling – a unique plan which really will provide you with a blueprint for healthy living for the rest of your life. It has been tried and tested by the most difficult, demanding panel of slimmers that I have ever worked with: the people of Fatfield, Tyne and Wear, England.

Many other diet books claim that they can provide the answer to every slimmer's prayers. And, it's true that any eating plan which cuts calories below the number required to maintain your body weight at your present level of energy expenditure will make you lose weight – that is if you can stick to it. The sad fact is that most overweight people cannot stick to a diet if it does not satisfy their longing for big, hearty, family-size meals. Facing a small helping of cottage cheese and a salad followed by a piece of fruit for lunch or supper may be fine for a week or so, but you would have to be a saint to follow such a depressing regime for very long. What's more, it certainly wouldn't be healthy to do so.

FOOD IS FUN
The Fatfield Diet is different from many other diets which seem to assume that slimmers want to suffer while they lose pounds. It works on the wicked principle that eating is life's second greatest pleasure. (No prizes for guessing what is life's top pleasure!) Food should be enjoyed, savoured, and eaten with delicious relish. Every meal should be a feast – from the sandwich you nibble alone at lunchtime, to the fabulous dinner you sit down to at Christmas or on some other special occasion. Food is comforting. Food is sexy. Food is social. Food is indulgent. Food is sensual. Food is wonderful!

Luckily, current nutritional thinking encourages a type of eating that goes along with these refreshingly greedy principles. Over the last few years, scientists and doctors have come up with a set of sensible guidelines which help you to eat more and weigh less. Although nutrition is a science which is evolving all the time, these ideas will stick around for many years because they have been proved to be healthy, thanks to a number of different controlled studies.

The main guidelines laid down by the scientists are that we should all cut back on fat and sugar, and increase the amount of fibre in our diet. It is particularly important to cut back on fat as this has been linked to heart disease so convincingly that the vast majority of doctors now accept it as fact. Sadly, people in this country still get an amazing 40 per cent of their daily calories from fat, which is why we have one of the highest incidences of heart disease in the world.

Sugar is highly addictive stuff because it provides a huge number of calories with virtually no other nutrients at all. We eat approximately about 2lb of sugar per person every week in this country; that is about 3500 calories which is enough for a whole day's meals for a man in a strenuous job. So, it is obvious that many overweight people can blame their 'sweet tooth' habit for at least some of their slimming problems. It makes sense therefore to cut down on sugar. On the Fatfield Diet you do just that but in such a way that you will never, ever feel deprived of your sugar 'fix'.

Fibre, which is found in fruits, vegetables, pulses like peas and beans, and grains, is a 'goodie' because it helps prevent diseases such as bowel cancer, diverticulitis, diabetes and heart disease. Foods containing plenty of fibre also have the advantage of being extremely filling so they figure strongly in the Fatfield Diet.

But, believe me, you won't have to go without meals like sausages and mash, burgers, and chips. You certainly won't be asked to give up delicious puddings, sweet snacks and treats, and you will not be eating so many fibre-filled baked beans that your friends wonder if you are following the F--Tfield Diet!

To help you turn meal times into the special occasions that they should be, we have devised dozens of tasty and filling recipes. They are very easy to make and all the ingredients are available from your supermarket. There are soups and starters, supper dishes, 'naughty' desserts and delicious snacks. Each recipe can be adapted to feed any number of people, from a large family to a single person. Of course each recipe has one special ingredient!

On the Fatfield Diet, every meal is a *whopping* great meal!

HOW TO FOLLOW THE DIET

Please do *not* start the diet until you have read all of Part One of this book. It will help your own slimming campaign to read all about the problems, occasional disasters and triumphs of our Fatfield guinea-pigs. The chapters on coping with your slimming campaign and finding motivation will provide invaluable inspiration. The exercise section will help you tone up while the pounds drop off. If the very thought of working out makes you feel limp and tired, don't worry. The Fatfield exercises are the easiest you have ever tackled. The only jogging you are asked to do is around the house, the only aerobics exercises are in a swimming pool so you do not feel the pain (or risk injuring yourself), and every work-out takes 20 minutes, or even less.

At the end of the book is a special section. Here there is a Calorie Guide to branded foods which I recommend for Fatfield slimmers. These have been selected for their nutritional value and appetite-appeal. In other words, they are tummy-filling, delicious and a useful addition to your shopping list. What's more, they have all been tested by a special panel of Fatfield food tasters and given top marks for scrumptiousness and value.

You will also find a Food Diary which I want you to fill in each day for a week, recording your meal intake, details of snacks, and how you coped with the diet. There is an address on page 121 where you can write with any problems you may have, and receive *free* advice from the Fatfield Diet slimming counsellors. If you want to be put in touch with a Slim Pal, for mutual support, full details are given too.

The most important thing of all is the Fatfield Charter. All slimmers should sign this before starting the diet. It is up to you whether you reveal your slimming ambitions to your family or friends. If you do decide to do this, pin the Charter on the kitchen wall for everyone to see. If you prefer to be a secret slimmer, keep the charter hidden away in a drawer, but DO sign it, as a constant reminder of your vow to stick to the plan.

Now, try the quiz below. It's fun, and also deadly serious, because it will help you to pinpoint approximately how many calories you are consuming right now. You could be surprised. Don't cheat!

HOW MUCH DO YOU REALLY EAT?

1. Which of these describes most closely your usual weekday breakfast meal? (Tick *one*)
    a) Cereal, milk, slice of toast and marmalade, tea or coffee
    b) Toast and a cup of tea or coffee
    c) Egg, bacon, sausage, beans, tea
    d) Nothing at all, or just a beverage

2. Which of these is most like your weekday lunch? (Tick *one*)
    a) Burger and chips
    b) Cooked meal in canteen or at home, such as chop and vegetables, pudding to follow
    c) Sandwiches and fruit or yogurt

d) Sandwiches and crisps
e) Pub lunch
f) Chinese or Indian takeaway
g) Salad with cheese, meat or fish

3. Which of these is most like your supper meal?
   a) Meat or fish and selection of vegetables
   b) Three course meal of soup, fish or meat, pudding
   c) Takeaway meal of fish and chips, Chinese, Indian, pizza
   d) Frozen ready-meal from supermarket
   e) Slimmer's ready-meal
   f) Snack meal: beans or egg on toast

4. Which of these between-meals snacks and confection-ary items do you eat? (Tick them *all* – no cheating!)
   a) About one packet of biscuits a day
   b) Up to four biscuits a day
   c) One or two bars of chocolate
   d) A few sweets
   e) A couple of slices of bread or toast and butter
   f) A scoop of icecream or iced lolly
   g) Bag of chips
   h) Slice of pizza

5. What is your daily alcohol consumption? (One unit is the equivalent of half a pint of beer or lager OR one pub measure short drink with a mixer, OR one glass of wine)
   a) 2 units, or less
   b) 2–4 units
   c) 4–6 units
   d) 6–8 units

6. What other drinks do you consume?

a) Tea or coffee with milk and sugar – 2 or 3 cups daily
b) Tea or coffee without sugar – 2 or 3 cups daily
c) Tea or coffee with milk and sugar – 3–6 cups daily
d) Tea or coffee without sugar – 3–6 cups daily
e) Tea or coffee without milk and sugar
f) Canned fizzy drinks – 1 or 2
g) Canned fizzy drinks – 2–4 daily

7. How much fruit do you eat?
a) 1 piece daily (eg. apple, orange, pear, grapefruit, slice of melon)
b) 2 pieces daily
c) 3 pieces daily

8. What are the main cooking methods used in your home? (Tick *one*)
a) Lots of fry-ups using fat or oil
b) Mainly grilling or roasting with a little fat added
c) Grilling, steaming, baking – no fat added

NOW ADD UP YOUR SCORE

	a)	b)	c)	d)	e)
1.	250	100	400	0	
2.	650	550	500	500	700
f) 1000	g) 300				
3.	450	650	1000	550	300
f) 350					
4.	800	350	500	350	300
f) 100	g) 350	h) 400			
5.	200	400	600	800	
6.	150	60	250	0	120
f) 140	g) 350				
7.	50	100	150		
8.	150	100	0		

The total will tell you, approximately, how many calories you are consuming each day. The average woman burns up around 2000 calories a day, and the average man between 2500–3000 calories.

It is very easy to exceed this total. For instance, if, on our quiz, you have ticked 1a, 2b, 3c, 4d, 5a, 6a, 7a and 8b your daily calorie total is just over 2500. This is fine if you are a man who wants to stay the same weight, but disastrous if you are a woman who wants to lose weight. In fact, with a pound of body weight being roughly equivalent to 3500 calories, you are probably putting on weight at the rate of around 1lb a week. Which might not sound much, but adds up to nearly 4 stone a year!

But, I promise you that is the very last sum you have to do. On the Fatfield Diet I have done all the sums for you. You will be cutting calories safely and easily while adding bulk and filling-power to your meals.

NOW GET RID OF GUILT

After completing the quiz above, you are probably feeling riddled with guilt about the amount you are eating and drinking.

Before you start reading more about the diet that *is* going to work for you, I want you to do something very difficult: stop feeling guilty – right now!

In twenty years of slimming counselling my assistants and I have helped thousands of people to reach their ideal weight. The biggest hurdle we have had to overcome has been guilt. Guilt is time-wasting, destructive, and fattening. It makes slimmers worry about their ability to stick to a diet, about being selfish while they are on the diet, and also about giving in during moments of extreme temptation. Every overweight person I have ever counselled – from politicians to pop singers – has felt guilty about their eating habits, particularly about their cravings for big, satisfying meals.

Why? Because we are all constantly being exposed to magazine articles, television programmes, and news reports about the dangers of overeating. At the same time, the opportunities for overeating have never been greater. Every high street has a wide range of fast-food restaurants and takeaways to choose from. Every supermarket has a huge selection of tempting goodies which make you long for an orgy of doughnuts, pasties and meat pies. It is humanly impossible *not* to be led astray. Yet, we *know* (or think we know) that it is wrong to indulge. No wonder most people are confused as well as guilt-ridden. It is *unfair*!

Let me give you a good example of the kind of person who is likely to be a victim of this guilt syndrome. She is approaching middle age, the mother of two teenage boys, works at a desk all day, and wants to provide a loving home and good, hearty meals for her family. Brought up in the lean, post-war years, she was always encouraged to clear her plate. She grew up in a home where money was limited, but everyone ate well. Foods like bread and dripping, mutton stew, and roly-poly pudding were often on the menu. By the time she reached her teens, she was decidedly chubby. In her twenties, she dieted to achieve the ultra-thin 'Twiggy' look, in her thirties she struggled to stay reasonably slim, while constantly trying out crazy diets: orgies of pineapple and melon; and mounds of meat and fish, ridiculous regimes which left her feeling tired and run down.

Now, in her forties, she has stopped fighting the inevitable, and started to eat huge meals again, just like she did as a kid. She is beseiged by temptation: takeaways, fast food, and restaurant meals. At the same time, she wants to be healthy, active and look good – knowing that women like Jane Fonda, Cher, and Raquel Welch look amazing in their forties and even fifties. Guilt? She is riddled with it!

This story is true, apart from the ending. The woman in question is *me*, and I am now eating more than I did as a teenager because I am following the Fatfield Diet. My weight is 8 stone 12lb, compared with 10 stone in my teenage days. I eat three huge meals each day, enjoy a daily alcoholic drink and I have never felt better in my life. Guilt is *not* on my menu! It doesn't have to be on yours.

CHAPTER TWO

THE FATFIELD
EXPERIMENT

When I first started writing about slimming back in 1974, high protein diets were frequently recommended. Doctors advised their overweight patients to stop eating bread and potatoes (incredibly, some still do) and eat plenty of steaks, fatty roasts and hard-boiled eggs. Not surprisingly, people developed bad breath, became constipated and got very bored while trying to slim down. In those days, it was fashionable for women to have an ultra-thin body. Many became ill in their quest to achieve the perfect shape.

Strange theories abounded: people latched onto any crazy eating plan that sounded as though it might work. They stuffed themselves with bananas and milk or ate a whole grapefruit without sugar before every meal, or even made themselves sick by taking amphetamine-related drugs. One particularly daft diet involved drinking a glass of wine for breakfast, then finishing up the bottle during the day, while eating nothing but salad. Fans of this crazy plan did sometimes lose a lot of weight, but they were usually too drunk to enjoy their new look!

At around that time, books and specialist magazines started to appear which examined the whole subject of losing weight in much more detail. Scientists discovered that we need more fibre in our diet, the links between high fat consumption and heart disease were explored, and the importance of trace elements and enzymes was revealed. A much healthier approach to dieting was encouraged. At the same time, various slimming clubs opened up. Each club had its own diet plan with group leaders (usually successful slimmers themselves) to help members to put it into action. The club method of slimming worked well, which is why it grew into the multi-million-pound business that it is today. However, some overweight people found that the often rigid approach of the slimming club could be off-putting.

While these publications and clubs educated people about a healthier approach to slimming, there were also some interesting new ideas on treating the psychological problems associated with obesity. At lectures and seminars, psychologists expounded their views on the 'new' ways to help people to slim successfully. We were told that 'comfort eating' was a peculiarly feminine problem which could only be solved if women became more assertive; 'dieting' was suddenly a dirty word! Then, behaviour therapy became popular. We were told that meals must be eaten at the right time, in the correct environment, and food must be chewed a certain number of times with a long pause between mouthfuls. It was all useful stuff, although sometimes taken to extremes, and often impractical.

As a reporter, I informed my readers about *all* of these fascinating things. But, they still wrote to me in their thousands wanting the perfect diet, and they were still willing to try almost anything in the vain hope that, this time, they had found it. Indirectly, their letters led to the creation and testing of the Fatfield Diet. Here's what happened.

Part of my job has always been to try out new products and diets for the special features I write. I never, ever recommend anything unless it has been tested thoroughly. It would be pretty simple to go along to a slimming club and let members try out a new diet product. But this would be a 'cop-out' because members have already taken the first step by joining the club, so they are primed to succeed. It is also cheating to test new diets and products on a group of highly motivated people who have easy access to healthy foods and lots of time to exercise. If they can't slim, who can?

I prefer to work with individuals or groups of people who find it very difficult to follow a diet because of the job they do, their lifestyle, or where they live. People with problems, people who work long hours, people who love eating.

Among the well-known people whom I have helped to slim are MP Emma Nicholson (who lost 20lb), Lord Prior (who lost $1^{1}/_{2}$ stone to raise money for Great Ormond Street Hospital), and comedian Frank Carson (who lost nearly 3 stone). The diets they followed were all created specially for them but included some elements which I later used for the Fatfield Diet. As ever, the most important rule for all three of them was to eat plenty so they never felt hungry.

Three years ago, I organised the first of my group slim-ins, helping 100 inhabitants of Broadbottom, a beautiful village near Manchester, to shed 100 stone in a month to raise cash for their annual carnival. The villagers love their food – and drink. So, it seemed rather dangerous to run the weekly weigh-in at the local pub. In fact, that turned out to be a splendid idea, as everyone could celebrate their weight-loss afterwards using up the generous alcohol allowance I gave them.

The Broadbottom experience convinced me that eating large meals while you slim down really works. Next, I moved on to an even more ambitious project, trimming eighty stallholders into shape at Tommyfields' Market, Oldham. This was quite a challenge, as the market is full of tempting fast-food stalls selling chips, mushy peas, pies and sausages coated in thick batter. But, again, the diet worked because our recipes were for filling, hearty dishes, and the stallholders lost 80 stone between them.

Next, it occurred to me that people who work for a brewery have special problems when it comes to losing weight. The draymen who load the kegs of beer onto the lorries, find that the work is heavy and thirst-making. The sales representatives who go out on the road spend their time sitting in bars discussing beer prices, surrounded by tempting snacks. Even those workers who stay in the office all day are in a thirsty environment, and everyone gets a daily beer allowance. My assistant, Toni Tompsett, told me about a group of workers at the Fremlin's Brewery near Maidstone in Kent, who were anxious to slim for the summer. We started working with them, and in less than six weeks, thirty slimmers had lost 30 stone between them. They shed the weight despite that beer ration. In fact, we did not ask them to give up alcohol and made sure that the menus were for large, family-size meals. Again, we were building up data and experience which, ultimately, contributed to the creation of the Fatfield Diet.

All this time, we were still replying to around 300 letters from readers each week, supplying individual advice, diet sheets, and contacts for specific problems. In addition, we organised phone-ins, so that people could ring up and talk to panels of experts, including nutritionists, doctors and fitness instuctors. This proved to be extremely popular and an excellent way of reaching those people who were too busy or too shy to join a slimming club. Where necessary, these phone-ins are followed up with mailed-out leaflets and diet sheets, all free of charge.

Then, the BBC asked me to help slim people working in jobs where it is particularly difficult to stay trim, for the popular daytime programme, 'Bazaar'. This is an excellent magazine-style show designed to help people who do not have a lot of spare cash. The hints and tips on everything from DIY to dressmaking are well thought-out and really do help viewers save money. The programme is screened on BBC-1 on Monday afternoons, and is repeated on Sunday mornings, from January to June.

We found two traffic policemen who were expanding rapidly because they spent so much time sitting in their police cars. We also took on a couple of lorry drivers who were putting on weight fast. In both cases, I provided a diet that fitted in with their lifestyles, including snacks to eat on the road and comforting meals to eat at home after a stressful day. In both cases, the weight-losses were excellent and the fitness levels attained by the four men were terrific. Once more, the one thing that made them all stick to the diet was that they ate so much food!

Last year, I suggested to 'Bazaar's' producer, Erica Griffiths, that we should try to help a whole community of people to slim down. I wanted to test out the 'eat more, weigh less' theory fully on a large group of people. The idea was to help them re-train their eating habits over the full six months of the series, from January to June 1991, with regular filmed progress reports. Again, I was adamant that these should *not* be people who were already committed to a slimming plan. I wanted a community where the local eating pattern was well-established and where the inhabitants enjoyed eating and drinking large amounts. We checked out several villages before we eventually decided to run the experiment in Fatfield, a village which is near Washington, Tyne and Wear, England.

The name of the village obviously had something to do with our choice, but there were also other important factors. First, the location of the village is extremely interesting: it nestles around the banks of the River Wear, about 15 miles from the port of Sunderland, close to the modern town of Washington, and around 8 miles from Newcastle-upon-Tyne. Fatfield marks the beginning of the River Wear Trail, a fascinating ramble along the banks of the river to Sunderland, tracing the history of the people who lived and worked there during the great nineteenth-century industrial explosion. Whole stretches of the river, once dominated by industry, have been returned to nature. Fatfield was once a flourishing mining village, but is now largely residential, with just three public houses, a couple of churches, a village school and two busy taxi firms.

I was struck by the fascinating history of the place. Legend has it that the famous Lambton Worm – really a dragon, and featured in the Geordie song of the same name – was finally slain at Fatfield after terrorising the neighbourhood by chasing sheep, killing cows and eating babies. The village grew from a series of smaller townships, chiefly inhabited by coalworkers. As long ago as the seventeenth century, it was a bustling industrial centre with a corn mill, an iron foundry and thriving businesses manufacturing coal tar, lamp black and coke.

Flat-bottomed boats based at Fatfield brought coal down the river to Sunderland for transportation to London. The 'keelmen' who piloted the boats, were such a huge, terrifying bunch that press-gangs looking for naval recruits avoided the area. By all accounts, the Fatfield people had a very hard life. The miners worked long hours in a dirty, dangerous job. Their wives worked equally hard, cooking hot meals throughout the day, and washing their men's dust-covered clothes. Most households included several men working at the pit, on different shifts, so the poor lady of the house had to get up at all hours, and put meals on the table throughout the day. It is not surprising that the people had huge appetites, filling up on local specialities like pies, dumplings, best beef, mutton, kneaded cakes, and black pudding.

These days, the village is a lot quieter, although it does have a thriving community and arts centre, enthusiastic religious congregations and lively social events at the three pubs, conveniently situated next to each other along the river bank.

But, the people still have huge appetites, which made them perfect for testing out my diet plan. They can shop at the excellent supermarkets in Washington which have an even bigger choice of food than many of the stores in the South of England. Pies, pasties, and dumplings are still just as popular as they were 100 years ago. In addition, villagers have the opportunity to eat the modern foods which so often contribute to overweight: chips, pizzas, Chinese and Indian takeaways, cakes, and confectionary.

On my first visit to Fatfield, I had lunch at the attractive Riverside Inn, and was astonished at the size of the meal. My huge, oval plate was piled high with a vast piece of fish in batter, an enormous mound of chips and an outsize portion of mushy peas, a local speciality made with dried peas flavoured with sugar. The calorie content of this plateful was around 1000, which is a lot for one meal. As I ploughed my way through it, I realised that if the eating programme (which I had already decided to call the Fatfield Diet) succeeded here, it would succeed anywhere.

CHAPTER THREE

HEARTY EATING IS HEALTHY EATING

Are you fed up with being told that you should eat less to be healthy? Relax. For once in your life, you are about to be told that you probably do not eat *enough*.

Mealtimes are, on the whole, enjoyable occasions and any diet plan which makes you *stop* enjoying your food should be avoided. If you have ever tried to slim down and failed miserably because you stopped looking forward to your meals, you will know what I mean. That awful, depressing feeling which comes over you when you know that your family will be sitting down to a delicious Shepherd's Pie, vegetables and a big pudding, while you fiddle around with a boring salad, is familiar to most people. You kid yourself that the sacrifice will be worthwhile when you are able, at last, to struggle into a size 12 dress, or if you are a man buy a pair of 34-inch-waist trousers. Sadly, you will probably start to expand again once you go back to eating normally.

The body is like a car: it needs regular injections of 'fuel', that is food, to run smoothly and efficiently. That means we should eat three times a day, or even more. We use breakfast, lunch and supper as a means of breaking up the day as well as replenishing our tummies. For most of us, these meals are associated with social activities as well as putting food into our mouths. You may not feel that you are particularly social at breakfast, but you probably eat the first meal of the day (if you do bother to eat it) while you talk to your family, scan the papers or open the post. At lunchtime perhaps you chat to work colleagues or listen to the radio. In the evening, you probably eat supper while you talk through the day with your partner, or watch television. In each case, you have combined eating with another activity, which makes it doubly important in your life. To my mind this is as it should be.

But, if eating is good for us, why is around 50 per cent of the population overweight? The answer lies in what we eat. Consider these two menus, eaten by one of our Fatfield slimmers, a lady in her mid-thirties with two children and a part-time job. The first menu is a typical example of the food eaten during a working day before she started following the Fatfield Diet. The second is very similar to the kind of daily menu she enjoys today. As you can see she is now eating *more* than she was before.

BEFORE DIETING
Breakfast: cup of tea with full-cream milk and 2 teaspoons of sugar
Mid-Morning: 4 digestive biscuits, cup of coffee with full-cream milk and 2 teaspoons of sugar
Lunch: Beefburger and chips, fizzy drink
Mid-Afternoon: slice of chocolate cake, cup of tea with full-cream milk and 2 teaspoons of sugar
Supper: lamb chop, chips, grilled tomatoes, individual fruit pie, $^1/_2$ pint of lager or a glass of wine, cup of tea with full-cream milk and 2 teaspoons of sugar

This menu does not appear to be excessively heavy. For a start, the lady had no breakfast and a fairly light supper. She experienced hunger pangs throughout the day, particularly just before lunch, and during the evening while watching television. She had tried to slim in the past by cutting out biscuits and chips, but somehow could never stick to this. The foods on the menu contain about 115 grams of fat, only 10 grams of fibre and approximately 2500 calories.

ON THE FATFIELD DIET

Breakfast: 1 cup of tea with skimmed milk and sweetener, 1 slice of wholemeal toast topped with 2 tablespoons baked beans, grilled tomatoes

Mid-Morning: 1 pear, 2 crispbreads topped with low-fat cheese, 1 cup of coffee with skimmed milk and sweetener

Lunch: 1 mug of slimmer's soup, large wholemeal sandwich with filling of salad, cold cooked chicken, 1 pear, 1 glass of mineral water

Mid-Afternoon: 1 low-calorie fruit yogurt, 1 cup of tea with skimmed milk and sweetener

Supper: Portion of Fatfield Shepherd's Pie, green beans, carrots, braised onion, baked apple stuffed with a few raisins, ½ pint of lager or a glass of wine, cup of tea with skimmed milk and sweetener

When she was shown this menu, our slimmer protested that she would never be able to eat all the foods listed. However, she soon became used to the additional bulk, and the weight simply dropped off. She lost 20lb in two months comfortably without being hungry or miserable. The foods on the menu contain about 60 grams of fat, 56 grams of fibre and approximately 1300 calories.

As you can see, the second menu is much lower in calories than the first. It also contains more fibre and less fat. With a calorie saving of around 1200 daily, this slimmer was able to lose weight easily, despite eating more food, in terms of bulk, than she had ever eaten in her life!

WHY CALORIES COUNT

Never believe any diet plan that tells you that you do not need to worry about calories. Sorry, folks, but I am afraid this is a big myth! Diets that tell you to eat certain foods at certain times of day, diets that preach that 'unlimited' amounts of meat and eggs will slim you down, diets that suggest alternating fruity days with indulgent days – they are *all* doomed to failure unless the basic sum (i.e. calorie intake must be *less* than calorie expenditure to produce weight-loss) is followed.

Especially dangerous are diets that consist of menus which do not specify exactly how much to eat. The authors are hoping that you will be so sick of a certain food, such as meat, that you will keep the amount to within sensible limits. In my work with thousands of slimmers, I know that nutritionists and dieticians often severely underestimate the ability of overweight people to consume huge amounts. While an 'average' 3oz (75g) portion of say, ham, only contains about 150 calories, some slimmers' ideas of an 'average' amount may be a half-pound of ham, thus adding 400 calories to the daily total. The *only* foods that you can eat freely on any diet (including this one – see page 35 for details) are leafy greens and salad vegetables which contain so few calories that you would have to stuff yourself silly to achieve a weight-gain if they were your only source of calories. The only drink that you can consume freely is water (which contains no calories at all). Diet soft drinks, black coffee and tea can, in theory, also be consumed freely, but too much of any of these is bad for your health and can affect, adversely, the success of your diet. Therefore, we do limit them on the Fatfield Diet.

So what is a calorie? The scientific definition is that it is the amount of energy needed to increase the temperature of 1 gram of water by 1 degree Centigrade. Sometimes, you see calories referred to as kilocalories. This is a more accurate name, really, because the kind of calories we are talking about would raise the temperature of 1 kilogram (i.e. nearly 2 pints) of water by 1 degree Centigrade.

If all that sounds like mumbo jumbo to you, don't worry. A much easier way of imagining what calories are is to think of them as, simply, units of energy supplied by the nutrients contained in food. The number of calories contained in a food depends on the kind of food it is. For instance, 1 gram of carbohydrate (in potatoes, bread, cereals, fruit) produces about 3.75 calories; 1 gram of fat (butter, lard, cooking oil, fat in meat) produces about 9 calories; 1 gram of protein (meat, eggs, fish) produces 4 calories and 1 gram of alcohol produces 7 calories. If you are measuring your food in ounces (as most people in the United Kingdom still are!), all you need to do is think of 100 grams as approximately 4 ounces. As you can see, foods which are high in fat produce the most calories, but 'booze' is pretty high too.

We 'spend' just over 1 calorie a minute merely to stay alive. That is, to maintain bodily functions such as breathing and digesting food. Once we do anything, sitting, walking, sleeping, exercising, the calorie expenditure increases accordingly. Of course, the total energy expended on any task depends not only upon the work involved but also upon the amount of energy the individual puts into it.

For instance, a very overweight person may be sluggish and droopy, even when performing simple tasks like walking around the house. On the other hand, they will certainly need to use up extra energy simply to move their bulk around from place to place.

So, calorie expenditure is a very individual thing, varying from person to person, depending on their lifestyle, weight, activities, and the amount of enthusiasm they put into them. Our daily calorie expenditure is also affected by some forms of medication (such as steroids and tranquillizers, which can make body metabolism and therefore energy expenditure sluggish), by changes in lifestyle (such as a change of job), by pregnancy and illness, smoking (and giving it up!) and even by emotional things like worry and falling in love.

However, the experts who have to decide what constitutes a healthy diet have given us guidelines to help us work out how many calories we need. As a rough guide, a woman in a sedentary job needs only around 2000 calories daily, a man around 2500.

This means that the vast majority of people can lose weight satisfactorily on 1500 calories daily. Certainly, women who are 2 or 3 stone overweight and most men should have no difficulty in shedding weight on a 1500 calorie diet. Women who have less weight to lose can do so very nicely on around 1200–1300 calories daily. *Unless* they have been putting their body into what we in the trade call 'starvation mode'.

This can happen when you have been following a diet that is very low in calories – usually *too* low. Since the human body is incredibly adaptable, it becomes used to this amount of nourishment each day. Your body 'decides' that you have probably been marooned in the desert with just starvation rations, or sent on a mission to the moon which has overshot, and food is running out. So, when you suddenly increase your calorie intake, your body conserves energy like crazy, laying down fat stores in case you are not rescued from the desert, or that mission to the moon. The best way to deal with this situation is to 'rev up' your metabolism by eating little and often, gradually increasing calories to a more sensible level, and stepping up exercise at the same time. The Fatfield Diet has a special plan for people who are experiencing this problem, which also works very well if you are stuck on a dieting 'plateau', where weight simply refuses to budge. If you have this difficulty check it out on page 76.

So, if calories matter so much, surely it is a good idea to throw away diet books, buy a good calorie counter and work out your own menus? Sorry, but NO! The problem here is that it can be all too tempting to 'spend' your daily calorie allowance on foods that you enjoy but do not do you much good. You then check your calorie total at lunchtime and find, to your horror, that you have already consumed 1500 calories in biscuits, sweets and soft drinks. There is nothing left for supper. Even if you have sufficient will-power and nutritional know-how to plan sensible meals, it is very fiddly indeed to work out exactly how many calories they contain, and you could fool yourself by leaving out things like cooking oil, drinks, and nibbles.

What *is* a good idea, is to start becoming 'calorie aware'. That is, to be canny enough to know which foods are high in calories and which are low. It means you should start looking at branded foods in supermarkets (many – although not enough – now give calorie values on the packaging), and checking out the list of Favourite Fatfield Foods on page 291. Our Fatfield slimmers have been doing some supermarket spot-checking and food-tasting themselves, and we have compiled a list of their favourite low-calorie buys. They have all been tested by our slimming team, and rated tops for value, taste and slim-power.

A final note on calories: there are very few people indeed who will not lose weight on a calorie-controlled diet. If you think you are one of these few, talk to your doctor before trying this, or any other diet. But first, keep a food diary for a week (*see* page 295), to make absolutely sure that you are not kidding yourself, and wasting your doctor's time.

FAT MAKES YOU FAT

Imagine a greasy, glutinous globule of fat. It is shiny, runny and looks absolutely disgusting as it disappears down the drain. It looks equally disgusting, hard and white, as it floats obscenely on top of leftover gravy. Now imagine it in your tummy, settling down gently on your stomach lining before being broken up by digestive juices and whisked away via your bloodstream . . . to block up your arteries or sit on your *hips*! Yuk.

Would you believe that we in Britain get an amazing 40 per cent of all our calories from *fat*? Yes, we eat the stuff voluntarily, as part of our daily menu! That 40 per cent consists of the 'hidden' fat in made-up meat products like pies and sausages, and the all-too obvious fat that clings to foods like chips, fried eggs, and takeaways. It also includes the fat in dairy products like cheese, full-cream milk and butter.

It is now widely accepted that the high incidence of heart disease in Britain is definitely linked to our appallingly high consumption of fat. So, it makes sense to cut fat for health reasons as well as to shed weight. However, it is not a good idea to try to cut out fat completely, as some diets suggest. Why? Because there are certain types of fat that are essential – even if only in small quantities – and some vitamins are present in fat (such as Vitamin D). It is also thought that polyunsaturated fats (in sunflower oil and oily fish such as herrings and mackerel) are good for your health. On the Fatfield Diet, these factors are taken into consideration.

But what about the taste of food? Does fat make it more palatable? For some people, heaven on earth is a greasy fry-up followed by a mug of milky coffee and a cream doughnut. If you are one of these, don't worry. Many of the original Fatfield slimmers thought that life would be grey and meaningless without greasy food. Honestly! Instead, they discovered that too much fat masks the real taste of chips, destroys the flavour of a cup of tea, and ruins the traditional British breakfast. Rather like giving up smoking, giving up eating so much fat gives your taste-buds a chance to savour food properly for the very first time.

SUGAR DOESN'T MAKE YOU SWEET
No, I am not going to give you another lecture on the subject of why sugar is bad for you. All I am going to say is that it contains absolutely nothing that does anything for your health or looks. There are no vitamins, minerals, fat or protein in sugar – just empty calories. About seventeen of them in every level teaspoon, a whole lot more hidden in foods like cakes, pudding, confectionary, many instant desserts, fizzy drinks and even canned vegetables.

Obviously, if you can cut back on sugar, you will cut back on calories. No, you will not go all weak and feeble if you stop having sugar in your tea because the body has ready supplies of glucose in the bloodstream and glycogen in the liver to spring into action when needed. No, it is not alright to replace ordinary, refined sugar with brown or demerara because they are just as fattening. If you are a honey fan, I am afraid that the bad news is that it is fattening too, although it has other properties which are beneficial.

On the Fatfield Diet, sugar is trimmed back as much as

possible. Which doesn't mean to say that you are not allowed to eat sweet foods. Fruits, puddings and some confectionary are permitted, but you must follow the diet-plans and recipes exactly.

PROTEIN: HOW MUCH DO WE NEED?

Protein, in meat, fish, eggs, cheese, and pulses such as beans, helps to build, maintain and repair the body. As I have already mentioned there was a time when high pro-tein diets were extremely fashionable. Nowadays, scien-tists believe that we probably do not need as much protein as was previously thought – especially if we are adults who no longer need to 'build up' our bodies.

Indeed, some diet doctors advocate substituting com-plex carbohydrate meals (potatoes, rice, pasta – not sugar, which is pure carbohydrate) for the traditional meat or fish and two-vegetable meal.

This is certainly one way of saving calories. As I men-tioned above, protein contains about 4 calories per gram, compared with 3.7 calories for carbohydrate. So if, for instance, you ate a jacket potato instead of a chicken leg with salad for lunch, you could save about 100 calories. If you normally ate the chicken leg with the skin on too, you would save even more.

However, while working with slimmers, I have found that eating some protein at each meal, in particular the first meal of the day, helps people to stick to a diet more easily. This is because protein definitely makes a meal more satisfying and prolongs that feeling of fullness. Protein foods 'burn' more slowly, sustaining energy levels for longer.

The problem is to find protein foods which are not bursting with fat as well. Cheese is definitely a dodgy one, since the protein it contains is mixed up with over half as much again in pure fat. Meats like pork and lamb are also dangerous for you can see the fat before your very eyes. Beef is possibly even 'naughtier', since the fat is often hidden in the flesh, giving just a slightly marbled effect to the meat. So, it is vital to look for very lean cuts and minced beef that contains only a small proportion of fat, and then to get rid of as much as possible during cooking. Even eggs are a problem as egg yolks are just about the fattiest thing you can eat apart from butter. In any case doctors now recommend cutting egg consumption to only four a week because of their high cholesterol content.

So which are the 'goodies' among the protein foods? They are fish, chicken (not the skin), low-fat yogurt, cottage cheese and pulses like baked beans, lentils and kidney beans. These foods are good sources of protein, so dishes containing them really do 'stick to your guts', and yet are low in fat, too.

On the Fatfield Diet, we have found ways of choosing and cooking other delicious protein foods to get rid of excess fat. We have also increased the protein power of cooked dishes by adding beans or yogurt. Many slimmers have slipped 'off the wagon' after having their nostrils assailed by the delicious smell of bacon sizzling away. That is one form of protein that you do not have to give up on the Fatfield Diet! Sounds good, doesn't it?

FIBRE: THE INCREDIBLE BULK

Do you want to feel full, instantly? Ignore those chocolate biscuits and crunch an apple instead. The reason apples are more satisfying than biscuits is because they contain fibre, so they take longer to chew. When each bit of apple reaches your tummy, the fibre absorbs water and you feel satisfied for ages instead of hungry again almost instantly.

So what is this magic stuff called fibre? It is the 'skeleton' or structural support that makes up all plants, from corn to cabbage. Although it does not contribute anything to our diet, it does help food pass through the body smoothly. A diet that is rich in fibre (in cereals, wholemeal bread, brown rice, wholemeal pasta, vegetables, fruits, bran) can help prevent diseases such as cancer of the bowel, diabetes, gall stones, diverticular disease and even heart disease.

In the West, we eat less fibre than people in Asia and Africa – around 20 grams a day compared with 50 grams. Scientists believe that we should try to increase our fibre intake to about 30 grams a day.

Fibre is incredibly useful stuff for slimmers . . . even if they do not like apples. Firstly, it helps make you feel full up without adding too many calories to your diet. That means you can sit down to a meal which includes a selection of fibre-rich vegetables (*not* boiled to death, which transforms the fibre into a mush) and get up from the table with a nicely satisfied tummy. Secondly, there is evidence that fibre 'chases' calories out of our bodies so they are not even absorbed. Although the number is small, around 5 per cent of the calories consumed, this is certainly a useful 'plus'.

The main disadvantages of adding too much extra fibre to your diet are the embarrassment of increased flatulence and the fact that it can prevent the absorption of minerals like iron and calcium. We must report that slimmers on the Fatfield Diet did *not* cause a sudden rush of wind through the Wear valley. Our diet is rich in fibre but not so rich that you will feel uncomfortable and lose all your friends as well as those much-needed minerals.

BIG IS BEAUTIFUL

If you use all the information above when you are planning everyday meals, you can in fact increase the size of those meals while reducing the number of calories they contain.

That is what we have done on the Fatfield Diet. Here are some examples of menus that apply to Fatfield principles. Read them through before you turn to the next chapter for your Basic Diet Plan.

BREAKFASTS

Non-Diet Meal: 3 slices toast and butter with marmalade, coffee or tea, milk and sugar. Calories: 400

Fatfield Meal: 1 bowl bran flakes and a little skimmed milk, 1 slice toast with low-fat spread, 1 size 3 egg, 1 apple. Calories: 350

Non-Diet Meal: 1 fried egg, fried bacon rasher, fried pork sausage, 1 slice fried black pudding, 1 slice fried bread, 1 slice toast and butter. Calories: 1090

Fatfield Meal: 1 rasher grilled bacon, grilled tomatoes, poached egg, 1 grilled low-fat sausage, 1 slice grilled black pudding, 2 slices toast, low-fat spread, 1 pear. Calories: 550

LUNCHES

Non-Diet Meal: 1 round cheese and pickle sandwich with butter, 1 meat pasty, 1 can cola drink. Calories: 635

Fatfield Meal: 2 rounds wholemeal bread and salad sandwiches with 1oz (25g) chicken, 2oz (50g) tuna, 1 Diet Ski yogurt, 1 can diet cola. Calories: 410

Non-Diet Meal: 1 Big Mac and chips, 1 cup of coffee with milk and sugar. Calories: 840

Fatfield Meal: 6 chicken McNuggets, huge mixed salad, 1 slice of melon, 1 mug slimmer's soup. Calories: 345

SUPPERS

Non-Diet Meal: untrimmed grilled pork chop, chips, mushy peas, trifle. Calories: 1500

Fatfield Meal: trimmed grilled pork chop, jacket potato, broccoli, cabbage, cauliflower, green beans, slice of Toni's Amazing Trifle. Calories: 550

Non-Diet Meal: Pâté and toast, scampi and chips, slice of Black Forest gâteau. Calories: 1400

Fatfield Meal: Clear soup, fillet steak and large mixed salad, jacket potato, lemon sorbet. Calories: 650

WHY YOU DON'T HAVE TO GIVE UP ALCOHOL

Any slimming counsellor will tell you that one of the quickest ways to lose weight is to give up alcohol. This is especially true for those men who normally drink a lot of beer. They only have to stop having 6 or 7 pints of lager or bitter every night to shed weight very rapidly indeed. They do not even have to stop eating fatty foods or sweets because alcohol is so high in calories that just cutting out one vice produces the required results, even if they carry on with their bad eating habits.

The sums speak for themselves: one half-pint of beer or lager contains about 100 calories (the same as a 'double' pub measure short drink, or a glass of wine). The increasingly popular strong lagers contain nearly *twice* that amount.

So, if a man is drinking 6 pints of beer a night, he is consuming at least 1200 extra calories, which is enough for a large meal. Over a week, that sum becomes a massive 8400 calories. With 3500 calories producing approximately 1lb of body weight, you can see that a chap can easily lose over 2lb a week by giving up drink.

The problem is that the vast majority of drinkers can only give it up for a short space of time, and then go back to drinking regularly. Result? The weight piles back on again.

On the Fatfield Diet I recommend drinkers to cut *back* on alcohol, but not to try and give it up altogether unless there are medical reasons for doing so. In my experience, it is more practical, and easier to cut down than give up. If you set yourself too many mountains to climb at any one time, you are much more likely to fail.

I must also say that, in my opinion, a certain amount of alcohol is *good* for you, particularly if it is in beer or wine rather than in spirits. The 'hard' stuff contains no vitamins or minerals, just 'empty' calories and it is all too easy to drink far too much of it, especially if you get into the habit of drinking spirits at home, where every tipple is a triple.

One of my favourite nutrition experts is the eminently sensible Dr Gaston Pawan, Senior Lecturer in Metabolism at the Middlesex Hospital Medical School in London. He has advised me for many years and has a refreshingly down-to-earth approach. Dr Pawan is one of the world's top authorities on alcohol and its effects on the human body. He believes, as I do, that drinking a modest amount socially is relaxing and helps to prevent stress, which is a major cause of heart attacks. He says, 'A couple of glasses of wine, or a pint of beer daily certainly won't hurt you. An occasional night out on the town with good company, a little good wine and lots of laughs is a far better tonic than anything your doctor can prescribe.' My own favourite drink is Guinness which I regard as a tonic as well as a delicious treat. It contains iron, Vitamin B and minerals, and contains about 100 calories in a half-pint measure. People often ask how I manage to stay slim and carry on drinking a pint of stout (sometimes more!) every day, but I simply make sure that I take the 200 calories into account on my Fatfield Maintenance plan. It is my treat, it does me good, and I make no apologies for enjoying every delicious sip!

CHAPTER FOUR

THE FATFIELD DIET: BASIC PLAN

The main principle behind the success of the Fatfield Diet is that slimmers *must* eat large, satisfying meals. Of our guinea-pigs from the village of Fatfield, the few who experienced difficulty sticking to the plan invariably had problems because they did not eat enough.

Remember: you will *not* lose weight any faster if you try to speed things up by eating less. You will only binge later on, making yourself feel guilty in the process. Don't do it!

Even if the amounts of food listed seem larger than you are used to, eat them up and enjoy them. I promise that you *will* become slimmer, healthier and feel wonderful.

The Fatfield Diet consists of a Basic Plan, plus eleven variations of this plan:

The Basic Fatfield Diet Plan   This is suitable for men, or women, who lead a fairly sedentary life. That's people like me who combine looking after a family with a sitting down job, or those who do light factory work or run a home full-time. However, it is *not* suitable for men or women with more than 4 stone or less than 7lb to lose. They should go for the Steady Weight Loss or Quick Weight Loss diets in the next chapter. Also, men in heavy, manual jobs, should choose the Heavy-Duty diet in Chapter Five.

The Eleven Variations   These cater for special needs and you will find them in the next chapter. They include plans for shift-workers, people who are in heavy, manual jobs, and vegetarians. In Fatfield, we found that these spin-off diets, together with the basic plan, provided a suitable diet for everyone. Where necessary, the plan was changed to cope with changing circumstances, such as a new job. Flexibility is vital while you slim. There is nothing wrong with switching plans mid-way. In fact, it can help give your metabolism a boost and prevent boredom, which is often the one thing that prevents slimming success. Never believe pundits who preach that you *must* stick rigidly to one diet, however limiting or boring it is – it just isn't true!

CONSULT YOUR DOCTOR BEFORE YOU START
No, this isn't the usual diet book 'cop-out' clause – it is sound common sense. These days, doctors are far more aware of the health problems associated with obesity and most surgeries now run some kind of preventive medicine plan such as regular health-screening sessions. So it is sensible to pop along to your doctor for a check-up before you try to lose weight. If you are very obese or are on medication for a specific problem, or are diabetic, it is absolutely essential to do so.

FREE VEGETABLE LIST: EAT AS MUCH AS YOU LIKE

There are certain vegetables which are so low in calories that you can eat them freely on the Fatfield Diet. Sounds like good news? Well, it certainly makes shopping a whole lot easier and it also helps you to enjoy the huge, hearty meals that are a vital part of the diet.

Why do we say this? Well, other diets sometimes tell you to measure out quantities of vegetables – 4oz (100g) of cabbage or a solitary tomato. But since cabbage contains only 6 calories an ounce, and tomatoes contain about 12 calories each, you would have to eat a lot of either to put on an ounce. So, what is the point of limiting them? What's more, vegetables contain fibre which fills you up and is good for you.

Where possible, shop for tasty fresh vegetables. Nutritionally speaking, frozen are just as good but there is often a great difference in taste. Watch out for tinned vegetables, though, since they sometimes contain additives such as sugar or salt. If you want to save cash while you slim, check out local markets for cheaper vegetables. But always make sure that they look fresh, since valuable vitamins (particularly Vitamin C) can be lost if vegetables are left hanging around for days on a market stall. Greens should be *green* not yellow. Tomatoes, peppers and beans should be firm to the touch.

Serve vegetables very lightly boiled, steamed or as huge, satisfying salads. Use garlic (helps reduce cholesterol in the blood, so is a 'goodie' in itself), herbs, lemon juice or vinegar to make a dressing (*see* Basic Salad Dressing recipe on page 172). Do *not* add butter or oil in cooking. Honestly, you will never miss that huge knob of greasy butter on your cabbage, but your hips *will* miss it, with great results.

Here's your 'free' vegetable list:

Asparagus	Chicory
Beansprouts	Chinese Leaves
Broccoli	Chives
Brussel Sprouts	Courgettes
Cabbage	Cucumber
Cauliflower	Curly Kale
Celeriac	Endive
Celery	Fennel

Gherkins
Leeks
Lettuce
Mushrooms
Mustard and Cress
Peppers (red and green)
Radishes
Runner Beans
Shallots
Spinach
Spring Greens
Spring Onions (scallions)
Tomatoes (tinned or fresh)
Watercress

TEN WAYS TO SERVE THEM
Remember: the bigger the portion size, the better!

1. *Make sensational tomato sauce.* Simply poach chopped mushrooms and finely chopped onions in a saucepan of tinned tomatoes, with herbs, garlic and lemon juice. Serve with meat, fish or even on toast as a snack.

2. *Discover the delicious taste of raw spinach.* Use spinach leaves, washed and lightly torn up as the basis for a fabulous salad. Just toss them with sliced raw mushrooms, chopped celery, sprigs of cauliflower, lemon juice, vinegar and seasoning.

3. *Make cauliflower exciting.* Divide it into florets, boil very lightly and serve with a topping of tinned tomatoes which have been mashed lightly and heated through with herbs and lemon juice. You can do the same thing with leeks or braised celery.

4. *Check out the different tomato varieties.* Grill large beef tomatoes as a tasty, supersized accompaniment to meat;

enjoy the sweet taste of tiny cherry tomatoes on salads; and use the long-shaped Italian tomatoes in cooking. They are all delicious.

5. *Try braising.* Some vegetables taste delicious if baked in the oven in a little chicken stock. Try braising whole chicory, leeks or celery in a shallow casserole. There is no need to put butter on the vegetables. They will cook beautifully without.

6. *Make enormous salads* – and eat them at any time. You can have four or five salads a day if you like, as well as all your Fatfield Diet foods. Try cooked, cold runner beans with spring onions, radishes and chopped gherkins or cucumber and tomato with strips of red and green pepper. Or, you can serve up a hot salad – a mixture of cooked, leftover vegetables, whirled through the microwave and topped with any Fatfield Salad Dressing.

7. *Go Chinese with beansprouts.* Use this delicious, crunchy vegetable as a hot vegetable. Tinned beansprouts are in every supermarket and are just as low in calories (about 3 an ounce) as the fresh variety. You could even try growing your own. They are particularly delicious mixed with whole button mushrooms which have been poached in water mixed with lemon juice.

8. *Be an asparagus lover.* Just a few asparagus spears, cooked and chopped, add a luxury touch to salads. You can often pick up a bundle of asparagus cheaply in markets. They make a wonderful starter – eaten with your fingers and dipped into a little dish of a Fatfield Salad Dressing.

9. *Try a Fatfield Stir-Fry.* You need absolutely no fat to make it since vegetables will sweat naturally. Just start by pouring half a tin of tomatoes into a non-stick pan. Chop

the rest of your vegetables and add to the pan gradually, cooking gently until just soft. Season to taste.

10. *Be a vegetable artist.* Experiment with different ways of serving up salads and vegetables, to give a really colourful effect. Try piling individual heaps of washed, chopped, raw vegetables on a large platter. Or make a vegetable casserole, topped with sliced tomatoes, to accompany the Sunday roast. Don't forget – serve LOTS!

MILK: TRIM WITH SKIMMED

The Fatfield Diet allows $\frac{1}{2}$ pint skimmed milk daily for your tea and coffee. If you haven't tried skimmed milk before, you will find that it is much lighter, and thinner in taste, than the full-cream variety. It also has all the protein and calcium of ordinary milk. Most people find that they quickly begin to prefer it. It is certainly a taste that is well worth acquiring in terms of calories saved. Full-cream milk contains over double the calories (about 400 calories a pint, compared with 200 calories for skimmed).

BREAD: WHOLEMEAL IS BEST

Where possible, it is best to eat wholemeal bread on the Fatfield Diet. This is because, weight for weight, wholemeal is slightly lower in calories than white bread. It is also high in fibre, so a slice of wholemeal will make you feel fuller than a slice of white. But, you can also substitute brown or granary bread if you like, or one of the fibre-enriched whites. But where one slice of bread is given, this refers to a medium slice from a large cut loaf, not a thick chunk from an uncut one.

PORTION SIZES

When portion sizes are stated on the diet, you must stick to them carefully. Some foods, such as cheese and meat, are very calorie-intensive, so adding just a few ounces or grams more can jeopardise your slimming success. A pair of kitchen scales is a very useful investment, so you can measure portion sizes accurately. For convenience, in the diet plans 1oz equals 25g.

COOKING THE FATFIELD WAY

On the Fatfield Diet, we aim to cut right back on fat, so obviously cooking methods are vitally important. One of our star slimmers, housewife Rose Irwin (read her success story in Chapter Six) used the diet as a great excuse to throw out all her old cooking pans and invest in a new set of non-stick ones: 'After having them for twenty years, it was time for a change,' she says. 'I had been using a couple of pounds of lard a week for roasting meat and potatoes, and now I don't use any at all which is good for our family's health as well as my figure.'

Here are ten tips for healthy cooking:

1. *Grill, don't fry.* From now on you're going to use your grill-pan instead of your frying pan. Make sure your pan has a grid, so meat can cook on top of the grid while any fat drips through the grid and can be disposed of afterwards.

2. *Skim off the fat.* When you're cooking casseroles, always skim off any fat before serving up the meal. If you prepare a casserole for supper the day before the meal, and store it in the refrigerator, it is very easy to whisk out any globules of fat using a slotted spoon before you re-heat it thoroughly in the microwave or oven.

3. *Buy lean mince.* It is not a good saving to buy cheaper, fatty minced beef. Instead, go for the leaner type, and pour off all the fat after browning it, before you add other ingredients. In a dish such as Fatfield

Shepherd's Pie, we even advise putting the cooked mince on absorbant kitchen paper to blot off excess fat before combining it with beans and stock.

4.   *Serve oven chips*. Yes, we really do allow chips on the Fatfield diet, but they are the oven kind *not* the deep fried kind. The calorie saving is considerable. Oven chips contain about 45 calories an ounce, compared with about 80 calories for medium, deep fried chips. The 'naughtiest' chips of all are crinkle-cut which have a high surface area which soaks up the oil, so the calories mount up to around 90 an ounce.

5.   *Invest in a super set of kitchen knives*. You will need them for trimming fat off chops, removing the skin from chicken, and slicing vegetables. Where possible, buy meat from the butchery department of your supermarket instead of ready-packed. Then, you can ask the assistant to trim the meat *before* he weighs it, saving you extra pennies.

6.   *Be an artful poacher*. Poaching – cooking food gently in water or stock – is an incredibly easy way of eliminating the need for added fat. For instance, mushrooms taste better and remain plumper if they are poached in water or a little chicken stock, and the calorie saving is enormous, about 60 calories an ounce. Or, try poaching an egg in a tin of tomatoes in a deep pan – you simply crack in the egg, taking care to keep it whole, and cook gently until both tomatoes and egg are cooked. Serve on a slice of toast for a quick and easy breakfast that only contains 200 calories.

7.   *Never add butter or margarine to vegetables*. If you are frightened of protests from butter-loving members of your family, put the butter dish on the table so they can help themselves.

8. *Try grilling 'roast' potatoes and parsnips.* The traditional Sunday roast is definitely on the Fatfield menu. One easy way to save loads of calories is to parboil potatoes and parsnips, brush them lightly with a little melted low-fat cooking spread and place under the grill. Turn the vegetables a couple of times during cooking to crisp them up all over.

9. *Serve no-fat gravies and sauces.* Fatty sauces tend to smother the flavour of food, as well as adding calories. So, go for thin gravy made from a stock cube, tomato juice and water, or one of our sauce recipes.

10. *Find creamy alternatives.* If you love cream in your cooking, there are lots of low-fat alternatives which you can choose instead. Try using low-fat natural yogurt (not the thick, Greek kind, which is higher in fat), or low-fat fromage frais.

CONVENIENCE COUNTS
No, you don't have to spend your whole day slaving over a hot stove to follow the Fatfield Diet. Convenience foods are recommended where they are suitable. Our Fatfield Team have tried and tested lots of different ready meals, packet soups, spreads and desserts, some aimed at slimmers, some not. Those they have found to be useful and delicious, are included in the diet.

EVERY PLAN IS MULTI-CHOICE
On most slimming diets the most limiting thing is the lack of choice. You are expected to eat a certain breakfast, lunch and supper on Day One, then another set menu on Day Two, and so on. On the Fatfield Diet, every variation gives a choice of breakfasts, lunches, suppers and treats, and it's up to you to pick the one you fancy.

This means that you get freedom and flexibility. You can go out and socialise, entertain friends, live a normal life. However, we do advise slimmers to vary their meal-choices as much as possible, so that they get their fair share of vitamins and minerals. Variety is the key to a healthy diet.

TREATS
You deserve a treat, so have one. Nearly every plan gives a list of treats to choose from. Make sure you don't go without these. Make 'treat-time' a bit special – when you're curled up with a book, watching television or just feel you need a boost.

TIMING
Eat meals when they fit into your lifestyle, bearing in mind that late-night suppers tend to stick around, on your hips! Don't leave long gaps between meals (fill them with 'free' vegetables, or a treat), and *do* make sure that you eat your breakfast meal as early as possible. If you simply can't eat it when you get up, pack it in a plastic container and take it to work with you so you can eat it during your first break. I do not belong to the school of slimming thought that advocates skipping the first meal of the day if you don't fancy eating it. You need a reasonable meal after eight hours of fasting to 'rev up' your body into top gear. If you miss it, you'll eat more of the wrong foods later on. Sorry!

BUY A FATFIELD PLATTER
To give your morale a pre-diet boost, buy yourself an extra large plate. A typical Fatfield Platter is oval, measures 18 inches (46cm) across and is designed to hold a *lot* of food. You may have something similar in your crockery cupboard which you are currently using as a vegetable plate. Amaze

your family by using it for your own main meals. Pile on the 'free' vegetables and salads to make sure the plate is well filled up. Then sit back and watch their faces . . .

WHEN TO START YOUR DIET

When you have read through this book and studied all the diet plans, select the one most suited to your needs. At the weekend, shop for the foods you will need for the first few days of the diet, then start it on a Monday. Weigh in the same morning, and then on subsequent Mondays. Do *not* weigh yourself more frequently (and, even as I write this, I know that you will ignore me!) because you'll get impatient and frustrated. Expect to lose more the first week, less on following weeks. This is quite normal as the first few pounds that come off are fluid, not fat. Remember: the more slowly you lose it, the better chance you have of keeping it off.

SLIM WITH A PAL

Our Fatfield slimmers had the support and help of the whole group. If you can find someone to slim along with you, it really does make the going easier. Your 'Slim Pal' can be a partner, relative or close friend. If you would like to join our Slim Pals register, do write to the address given at the end of Chapter Seven.

BASIC PLAN – RULES

EVERY DAY   You may have $^1/_2$ pint (275ml) skimmed milk for your tea and coffee, unlimited water, mineral water and diet soft drinks. Use an artificial sweetener such as Hermesetas. No sugar is allowed.

However, I would advise slimmers not to overload their system with too many fizzy drinks, diet or not. The very best drink is the still kind of mineral water which is truly delicious served with ice and lemon. Drink LOTS.

MEN   You should add 1 extra slice of wholemeal bread or a medium wholemeal roll with a little low-fat spread, 1 apple, orange or pear and 1 extra glass dry wine or $^1/_2$ pint beer or lager to your daily total.

FREE VEGETABLES   Choose them from the list on page 35. Eat plenty!

CALORIES   The diet contains about 1350 calories daily for women, 1600 for men. This may sound a lot compared with other diets, but you want the weight to stay off, don't you? It *works*, honestly.

BREAKFASTS (choose *one*, packed if necessary)

- $^1/_2$ grapefruit, with sweetener, 1oz (25g) bran cereal with a little extra milk, 1 slice wholemeal bread with 1 tbsp honey

- 1 slice wholemeal toast with small can (5oz/125g) baked beans, small banana

- 2 Weetabix biscuits with milk from allowance, 1 apple or pear, slice of wholemeal toast with scraping of low-fat spread

- 2oz (50g) unsweetened muesli with milk from allowance, topped with 1 chopped apple

- 1 size 3 egg on 1 slice wholemeal toast, grilled tomato, 1 orange

- Sandwich of 2 slices wholemeal bread with filling of salad and $^1/_2$oz (12g) Edam cheese

- Medium wholemeal roll with filling of 1 rasher of well-grilled streaky bacon or 2oz (50g) cottage cheese, 1 apple or pear

- 1 mug Batchelors Slim a Soup, 2 crispbreads with scraping of Marmite, tomatoes, 1 large banana, 1 carton Diet Ski yogurt

LUNCHES (choose *one*)

Sandwich made with 2 slices wholemeal bread or a medium sized wholemeal or granary roll with one of the following fillings and accompaniments:

- Salad (from 'free' list), $^1/_2$oz (12g) Edam cheese, Diet Ski yogurt and 1 orange

- Salad and $3^1/_2$oz (88g) can tuna fish (canned in brine only, not oil), 1 small banana

- 1oz (25g) lean ham, 1 mug Batchelors Slim a Soup, large mixed salad from 'free' list, 1 apple

- 1oz (25g) chicken (no skin), large mixed salad, 4oz (100g) carton Shape Coleslaw Salad, 1 orange

OR
One meal from this list:

- 1 well-grilled beefburger in a wholemeal roll, large mixed salad, 1 small banana

- 2 slices wholemeal toast topped with small can (5oz/125g) baked beans and 1 size 3 poached egg, watercress, mixed salad

- 6oz (150g) jacket potato topped with 4oz (100g) chopped cooked chicken mixed with 1 tbsp low-calorie salad cream, 1 apple

- 1 large slice of melon, 10oz (250g) chicken leg (no skin), grilled or roast, huge mixed salad or vegetables from 'free' list, 1 small wholemeal roll with a little low-fat spread

- 6oz (150g) any grilled or steamed white fish (e.g. cod, sole, plaice), with no fat added, 5oz (125g) jacket potato, 1oz (25g) scoop vanilla icecream with 10 grapes

Don't forget to pile on the 'free' vegetables and salad.

SUPPERS (choose *one*)

- 5oz (125g) lean pork chop or tenderloin, Fatfield Bubble and Squeak

- Steak and Kidney Casserole, 8oz (200g) jacket potato, 1 apple

- Fatfield Shepherd's Pie, 4oz (100g) peas, ½ pint (275ml) custard (made up with skimmed milk and sweetener to taste added after cooking), and 1 small banana

- Pork Paprika, 6oz (150g) jacket potato

- McCain Cheese and Tomato Deep 'n Delicious pizza, 1 apple and 1 pear

- Liver and Onion Gravy, 6oz (150g) jacket potato, 2oz (50g) peas

- Bird's Eye Cod Steak in Wholemeal Crumb, 3 oz (75g) mashed potato, 3oz (75g) peas, 1oz (25g) scoop vanilla icecream, 1 small banana

- Piquant Mince with Dishy Dumplings, 6oz (150g) jacket potato, 1 satsuma or small orange

- $^1/_2$ grapefruit with sweetener to taste, 3oz (75g) any lean roast meat, thin gravy, 3oz (75g) large chunks roast potatoes or parsnips, 4oz (100g) carrots, 3oz (75g) peas, Toni's Amazing Trifle
- 5 fl oz (125ml) chilled apple juice, Crunchy Wholewheat Lasagne, 1 Diet Ski yogurt
- 6oz (150g) any white fish, grilled or steamed with a little low-fat spread (e.g. Gold Lowest) added, 10oz (250g) jacket potato, 1 apple or orange
- Indian Takeaway or Restaurant meal of Chicken Tandoori, plain boiled rice, onion rings, $^1/_2$ pint lager
- Chinese Takeaway or Restaurant meal of Chicken Chop Suey, plain boiled rice, 1 glass dry wine
- Steak House meal of lean fillet steak, jacket potato (no butter or soured cream), peas and 1 glass dry wine

Don't forget to pile on the 'free' vegetables and salad.

TREATS (choose *two* each day)
- 1 wholewheat crispbread topped with 1oz (25g) cottage cheese and scraping of Marmite
- 10 grapes
- 2 sticks celery with filling of 1oz (25g) low-fat cream cheese
- 1 apple or orange
- 1 medium digestive biscuit
- 1 mug Batchelor's Slim a Soup with 1 Ryvita crispbread

ALCOHOL ALLOWANCE
Every day, you are allowed $^1/_2$ glass dry wine *OR* $^1/_2$ pint beer or lager (if you are teetotal, you can have two 5 fl oz (125ml) glasses of unsweetened orange juice or tomato juice instead of these alcoholic drinks).

CHAPTER FIVE

DIET PLANS

Here are eleven diets, based on the Fatfield principle of 'Eat More, Weigh Less' to cater for those slimmers with special needs. They range from a Vegetarian Plan, to an Anti-Bloating Plan created for women who suffer from fluid retention caused by menopausal or pre-menstrual problems. Men can choose from plans like the Boozers' Plan, the Heavy-Duty Plan and the Shift-Workers' Plan.

If you live alone you will love the Lazy Cook's Plan which offers a super selection of easy-to-cook dishes, and includes some of the excellent ready meals available from your local supermarket.

A CHANGE IS AS GOOD AS A FEAST!

If you wish to change your diet during your slim-in, do so. But first, make sure that the plan you are switching to is suitable for your lifestyle and starting weight.

Don't forget to vary your meal choices so you get a good variety of nutrients.

QUICK WEIGHT LOSS PLAN

This is *only* suitable for female slimmers who have half a stone, or less, to lose. It is perfect for women who want to shed weight rapidly for a holiday or special occasion. Stay on it for a maximum of two weeks, then go on the Basic Fatfield Plan for more steady weight loss. Portion sizes are particularly important on this diet plan, so do invest in some kitchen scales if you can. Don't forget to nibble away at your 'free' salads and vegetables between meals. The more you eat, the more likely you are to stick to the diet.

You can swap lunch meals with supper meals if you wish.

EVERY DAY $^1/_2$ pint (275ml) skimmed milk for your tea and coffee, unlimited water and mineral water. Use artificial sweeteners only.

MEN Sorry, this diet is not for you.

FREE VEGETABLES Choose them from the list on page 35. Eat plenty!

CALORIES About 1000 calories daily.

BREAKFASTS (choose *one*, packed if necessary)
- 1 slice wholemeal toast with scraping of low-fat spread, 1 apple or pear
- 1 Diet Ski yogurt, any flavour, 1 large banana
- 1 size 3 egg, boiled or poached, 2 Ryvita crispbreads with scraping of low-fat spread
- 1oz (25g) any unsweetened cereal, milk from allowance, chopped apple on top
- small wholemeal roll with filling of 1 rasher well-grilled streaky bacon and grilled tomatoes
- 2 slices Nimble bread with filling of salad and 2oz (50g) cottage cheese

MID-MORNING SNACKS (choose *one*)

- 1 apple or pear
- 1 mug Batchelors Slim a Soup
- 1 Jaffa Cake

LUNCHES (choose *one*, again packed if you like)

Sandwich of 2 slices wholemeal bread with 'free' salad plus one of the following fillings and accompaniments:

- 1oz (25g) Edam cheese, 1 small banana
- 1 small jar of Shippams Beef or Fish Spread, 1 satsuma
- 2oz (50g) cottage cheese with chives and onion, a few grapes

OR

One meal from this list:

- Well-grilled beefburger in a bun (no onions) with 1 tsp relish, 1 orange
- Slimmer's Vegetable Broth, 1 wholemeal roll with a little low-fat spread and 1 Kraft Cheese Triangle
- 1 mug Batchelors Slim a Soup, $3^{1}/_{2}$oz (99g) tin tuna, canned in brine, 1 medium wholemeal roll with a little low-fat spread
- 1 slice wholemeal toast topped with small can (5oz/ 125g) baked beans, grilled tomatoes, 1 medium banana
- Citrus Salad in Yogurt Dressing, 10oz (250g) chicken leg (no skin), 1 apple or orange
- 7oz (175g) jacket potato with one of these toppings: 3 tbsp baked beans, 1 carton Shape Coleslaw Salad, 1 carton Shape Cottage Cheese, 2oz (50g) cold, cooked chicken mixed with 1 tbsp low-calorie mayonnaise,

3$^{1}/_{2}$oz (99g) tuna in brine mashed with lemon juice and a little vinegar

SUPPERS (choose *one*)

- 3 fish fingers, grilled with grilled tomatoes, 3oz (75g) mashed potato, 1oz (25g) scoop vanilla icecream
- 3oz (75g) lean roast meat, thin gravy, 3oz (75g) chunks of roast potato, 1 Shape Fromage Frais or Shape yogurt
- 3oz (75g) lean boiled ham or gammon, 4oz (100g) tinned pease pudding, 3oz (75g) potato mashed with some of the cooking liquid, $^{1}/_{4}$ pint (150ml) Bird's Sugar Free Jelly, 1oz (25g) vanilla icecream
- Fatfield Bubble and Squeak, 1 apple
- Fatfield Shepherd's Pie, 1 satsuma
- 1 large slice melon, Spaghetti Carbonara, 1 medium banana
- Liver with Onion Gravy, 2oz (50g) potato mashed with a little skimmed milk
- Mixed grill: 1oz (25g) black pudding grilled, 1 well-grilled beefburger, 1 well-grilled low-fat sausage, grilled tomatoes

Pile on the 'free' vegetables!

STEADY WEIGHT LOSS PLAN

This plan gives an excellent weight-loss for women who have 3 stone, or more, to lose, and men who have just a small amount of weight to shed. In Fatfield, several couples followed this plan together. It is also suitable for teenagers who want to lose a bit of weight safely. Make sure you eat your treats. The alcohol allowance is, of course, optional!

EVERY DAY   You may have $^1/_2$ pint (275ml) skimmed milk for your tea and coffee, unlimited water, mineral water and diet soft drinks. Use an artificial sweetener.

FREE VEGETABLES   Pile them on, choosing from the list on page 35.

CALORIES   About 1500 daily.

BREAKFASTS (choose *one*)
- 1oz (25g) any unsweetened cereal with milk extra to allowance, 1 slice wholemeal toast with 1 tsp jam or marmalade
- 5 fl oz (125ml) unsweetened fruit juice, 5oz (125g) can baked beans on 1 slice wholemeal toast
- 2 well-grilled rashers of streaky bacon, 1 slice wholemeal toast, 1 apple or pear
- $^1/_2$ grapefruit with artificial sweetener to taste, 1 size 3 egg, poached or boiled, grilled tomatoes, 1 slice wholemeal toast with a little low-fat spread
- 2 Weetabix, milk from allowance, 1 slice wholemeal toast, 1 tsp jam or marmalade, 1 Diet Ski yogurt
- Sandwich of 2 slices wholemeal bread, Marmite and 2oz (50g) cottage cheese

LUNCHES (choose *one*)
Sandwich made with 2 slices wholemeal bread or a crispy roll with any of the following fillings and accompaniments:
- 1 jar Sutherland's fish paste, 1 orange
- 1oz (25g) Edam cheese, 1 dsp pickle, salad, tomato, 1 satsuma

- 1 well-grilled low-fat sausage, 1 tsp tomato ketchup, 1 mug Batchelors Slim a Soup, 1 apple
- $3^{1}/_{2}$oz (99g) tuna, canned in brine, 1 tsp low-calorie seafood dressing, 1 apple
- 2oz (50g) cold chicken (no skin), diced and mixed with $^{1}/_{2}$ apple and 1 tbsp low-calorie salad cream, 1 Diet Ski yogurt
- 1 small carton cottage cheese with 1 ring chopped pineapple, 1 apple

OR

One meal from this list:

- 7oz (175g) can macaroni or ravioli, 1 slice toast, grilled tomatoes, 1 apple
- 2-egg omelette made in a non-stick pan with $^{1}/_{2}$oz (12g) low-fat cooking spread, 2oz (50g) lean ham, 1 mug Batchelors Slim a Soup
- Spaghetti Carbonara
- 10oz (250g) grilled chicken leg (no skin) with Barbecue Sauce, 1 orange or apple
- 1 Beefburger in a bun (no onions), 1 small banana
- 1 10oz (250g) jacket potato, with topping of 2 tbsp baked beans or 3 tbsp cottage cheese, 1 apple or orange

Pile on the 'free' salads and vegetables.

SUPPERS (choose *one*)

- 3oz (75g) lean, cold roast meat, 7oz (175g) jacket potato, $^{1}/_{2}$oz (12g) knob low-fat spread, 1 frozen mousse
- Piquant Mince, 4oz (100g) peas, 7oz (175g) potato mashed with some of the cooking liquid, 1 Shape yogurt

- 4 fish fingers, grilled, with grilled tomatoes, 7oz (175g) jacket potato, 4oz (100g) peas, 1 apple
- Fatfield Shepherd's Pie, 4oz (100g) peas, ½ pint custard (275ml) made with skimmed milk and artificial sweetener to taste, 1 small banana
- Aubergine Casserole, 6oz (150g) jacket potato, 1oz (25g) vanilla icecream, 2 peach halves, canned in juice or water
- Greek Vegetable Soup, 3oz (75g) any lean roast meat, thin gravy, 3oz (75g) roast potato, 3oz (75g) peas, 1 Diet Ski yogurt
- Bird's Eye Cod Steak in Wholemeal Crumbs, 3oz (75g) McCain oven chips, 1 apple or pear

Don't forget those 'free' vegetables.

OR *one* of these restaurant or takeaway meals:
- One portion Kentucky Fried Chicken with Coleslaw
- Chicken Tandoori with plain boiled rice
- Melon, 5oz (125g) fillet steak, 1 scoop vanilla icecream

TREATS (choose *two* each day)
- 1 slice wholemeal toast topped with Marmite or a little low-fat spread
- 1 fun size Mars or Snickers Bar
- 1 packet low-fat crisps
- 1 After Eight Mint and 1 small banana
- 1 mug of Batchelors Slim a Soup and 2 crispbreads with a little low-fat spread

ALCOHOL ALLOWANCE
You may have one glass of dry wine or $^1/_2$ pint beer or lager each day, or save it up for a night out. If you wish,

you may substitute *one* of your daily treats for another ration of alcohol

ANTI-BLOATING PLAN

Just before a period, or during the menopause, many women experience unpleasant bloating. This is caused by hormonal activity in the body. It has been found that cutting back on refined carbohydrate foods (cakes, sugary cereals) and salty foods (bacon, canned soups, nuts, kippers) can help reduce this unpleasant symptom. Cutting down on cups of tea and coffee can also help. Certain foods, notably citrus fruits and cucumbers, can help 'chase' the water away.

This plan follows the Fatfield principles. It is marvellous for PMT sufferers and super for menopausal women. Several of our Fatfield slimmers switched to this plan for one week every month, just before their period.

EVERY DAY   You may have $^1/_2$ pint (275ml) skimmed milk for your tea, coffee and cereals. Limit cups of tea and coffee to 2 a day, and make sure coffee is decaffeinated. Other drink options include herb teas and mineral water (serve chilled, with a slice of lemon). Try to drink more water than normal, about 6 glasses daily.

FREE VEGETABLES   Choose them from the list on page 35, and be liberal with lemon juice when you are making salad dressings.

NB Use salt-free stock cubes to make gravy. Do not add salt in cooking. Instead, just put it on the table so the rest of your family can help themselves. You will find that the meals are tasty enough not to need the addition of salt.

CALORIES   About 1200 daily.

BREAKFASTS (choose *one*)

- $^1/_2$ grapefruit with a little artificial sweetener (leave it out if you possibly can), 1 size 3 boiled egg, 1 slice wholemeal toast

- 1oz (25g) unsweetened cereal, milk from allowance, 5 fl oz (125ml) unsweetened orange juice, 1 apple or pear

- 5 fl oz (125ml) unsweetened grapefruit juice, 1 carton natural yogurt with chopped apple and a few raisins

- 4oz (100g) reduced-sugar and salt baked beans on 1 slice wholemeal toast, grilled tomatoes

MID-MORNING

- 1 piece fresh fruit (choose from 1 apple, orange, pear or small banana, 1 large slice of melon or 2 plums), 1 Diet Ski yogurt

LUNCHES (choose *one*)

- 7oz (175g) jacket potato with $3^1/_2$oz (99g) tuna, canned in brine, lemon juice, 1 orange

- Sandwich of 2 slices wholemeal bread, lemon juice, 2oz (50g) chicken or turkey (no skin)

- 5 fl oz (125ml) unsweetened orange juice, 2 crisp-breads with cucumber slices and 4oz (100g) cottage cheese, 1 apple

- 2-egg herb omelette cooked in a non-stick pan with $^1/_2$oz (12g) low-fat cooking spread, 1 Diet Ski yogurt

MID-AFTERNOON

- 1 Shape Fromage Frais, 2 crispbreads

SUPPERS (choose *one*)

- 3oz (75g) cold lean roast meat, 3oz (75g) mashed potato, made with milk from allowance, baked apple with filling of 2oz (50g) raisins, 1 crusty wholemeal roll.

- 5 fl oz (125ml) unsweetened orange juice, 6oz (150g) any white fish cooked in the oven in foil with lemon juice, sliced onion, sliced tomato, herbs, 7oz (175g) jacket potato

- 4oz (100g) grilled liver with sauce made from thin gravy and juice of 1 orange, watercress, 3oz (75g) boiled potatoes, 1 apple

- 4oz (100g) lean mince cooked 'dry', drained of fat and mixed with 1 small tin tomatoes, herbs and garlic to taste, 2oz (50g) (dry weight) pasta, 3oz (75g) raspberries with 1oz (25g) icecream

- 5oz (125g) lean lamb or pork chop, thin gravy, 3oz (75g) mashed potato, made with milk from allowance, a few grapes

- 3oz (75g) any lean roast meat, thin gravy, 2oz (50g) roast potatoes, 1 sliced orange with 2 chopped dates and a little lemon juice on top

- Fish Casserole, salad from 'free' list with Basic Salad Dressing, 1 orange

- 8oz chicken leg, skinned and casseroled in 1 can slimmers chicken or tomato soup, 1 crusty roll, a few grapes

ALCOHOL ALLOWANCE
You may have 1 glass dry wine or $1/2$ pint beer, lager or stout daily.

HEAVY-DUTY PLAN

This diet is suitable for men in heavy, outdoor work or fairly tough factory work indoors. It will help you slim down safely without feeling low or tired at work. The lunches can be packed or chosen from the canteen menu. If you prefer to go to the pub at lunchtime, there is a selection of meal choices for you. There is, of course, a daily alcohol allowance.

EVERY DAY   You may have $^1/_2$ pint (275ml) skimmed milk for your tea and coffee, unlimited water, mineral water or diet soft drinks. Use sweeteners instead of sugar.

FREE VEGETABLES   Choose them from the list on page 35. Pile them up on your plate.

CALORIES   About 1800 daily.

BREAKFASTS (choose *one*)

- 5oz (125g) can baked beans, 1 size 3 egg, 1 slice toast
- $^1/_2$ grapefruit, $1^1/_2$oz (38g) any unsweetened cereal with milk from allowance, 1 slice wholemeal toast with scraping of marmalade
- 1 size 3 poached egg, 1 rasher well-grilled back bacon, grilled tomatoes, 1 slice wholemeal toast
- 1 well-grilled low-fat sausage in a small crusty roll with tomatoes
- 2 rashers well-grilled streaky bacon, grilled tomatoes, mushrooms poached in water, 1 slice wholemeal toast
- 2 Weetabix or 2 Shredded Wheat with milk from allowance, 1 apple, 1 small banana

LUNCHES (choose *one*)

Packed Lunches (don't forget to add plenty of salad from your 'free' vegetable list):

- 2 crusty wholemeal rolls with 2 grilled chipolata sausages, 1 dsp sweet pickle, 1 apple
- 1 medium Scotch egg, 1 small wholemeal roll, 1 satsuma
- 1 bap spread with mustard, 2oz (50g) lean ham, 1 packet low-fat crisps, 1 orange
- 2 slices wholemeal bread with one of these fillings and accompaniments:
  - 1oz (25g) lean ham, 1 Diet Ski yogurt
  - 1oz (25g) Edam cheese, 1 apple or orange
  - 2oz (50g) Shape Low-Fat soft cheese, chopped gherkins, 1 carton Shape Fromage Frais

Canteen lunches (ask for a large side salad *and* a big portion of green vegetables with your meal):

- 10oz (250g) grilled chicken leg, small portion apple crumble
- Lamb or beef hot pot, 1 low-calorie yogurt or a piece of fruit
- 4oz (100g) mixed cold meats, 10oz (250g) jacket potato

Pub lunches (please ignore the Shepherd's Pie, pasta dishes and curries on display – they are invariably fat and calorie loaded, sorry!):

- Ham or chicken salad, 3in (8cm) slice crusty French bread, 2oz (50g) hard cheese
- Small portion quiche, large mixed salad, 1 apple or orange
- Scampi-in-a-basket, 1 dsp seafood dressing, large mixed salad

SUPPERS (choose *one*)

- 3oz (75g) cold, lean roast meat, 7oz (175g) jacket potato, $^{1}/_{2}$oz (12g) low-fat spread, 1 frozen mousse

- Piquant Mince with Dishy Dumplings, 4oz (100g) peas, 5oz (125g) potato mashed with milk from allowance, 1 apple

- Mixed grill: 4oz (100g) kidney, grilled tomatoes, 1 rasher grilled back bacon, 1oz (25g) grilled black pudding, 4oz (100g) mashed potato browned in $^{1}/_{2}$oz (12g) low-fat cooking spread, 2oz (50g) peas

- 4 grilled fish fingers, grilled tomatoes, 4oz (100g) McCain oven chips, 4oz (100g) peas, 1 apple

- Fatfield Shepherd's Pie, 4oz (100g) peas, ½ pint (275ml) custard made with skimmed milk and sweetener to taste, 1 small banana

- 4oz (100g) any lean roast meat, mini Yorkshire pudding made in non-stick tin, thin gravy, 3oz (75g) roast potato, 2oz (50g) peas, 1oz (25g) scoop icecream, $^{1}/_{4}$ pint (150ml) Bird's Sugar Free Jelly

- 5oz (125g) lean pork chop, Fatfield Bubble and Squeak

- 1 small Bowyer's Cornishman's Pasty (5oz/125g), 4oz (100g) potato mashed with milk from allowance, 2oz (50g) peas

- Steak and Kidney Casserole, 8oz (200g) jacket potato, 1 apple

OR

One of these Restaurant and Takeaway meals:

- 1 portion Kentucky Fried Chicken, coleslaw, barbecued beans, 1 apple or pear

- 6oz (150g) grilled rump or sirloin steak, fat removed, 8oz (200g) jacket potato, 2oz (50g) peas, 1oz (25g) scoop vanilla icecream
- Tandoori Chicken, plain boiled rice, 2 poppadums, 1 apple or pear
- Half a thin, medium pizza with vegetable and ham topping (NOT cheese!), huge mixed salad from salad table (avoid items with oily dressings), 1oz (25g) scoop vanilla icecream

TREATS (choose *two* each day)
- 1 fun size Mars or Snickers bar
- 2 digestive biscuits
- 1 crusty roll with a little low-fat spread
- 2 fingers of Kit Kat
- 1 packet low-fat crisps

ALCOHOL ALLOWANCE
You may have 2 glasses dry wine or 1 pint beer, lager or stout every day.

BOOZERS' PLAN

This diet will help most women, and all men to lose weight effectively. It allows some extra alcohol each day, which you can save up for one or two naughty nights out each week if you like. Sorry, it is *not* a drink-as-much-as-you-like diet! Try to make sure that you really enjoy the booze that you do have. If you are a lager drinker with a big thirst, it is always a good idea to have a refreshing low-calorie soft drink or glass of water before your first half-pint of booze, because the first drink just doesn't 'touch the sides' as it goes down.

EVERY DAY   ¹/₂ pint (275ml) skimmed milk for your tea and coffee, unlimited water and mineral water. Use artificial sweeteners only.

FREE VEGETABLES   Choose them from the list on page 35. Eat as much as you can.

CALORIES   About 1500 daily.

BREAKFASTS (choose *one*)

- 1 slice wholemeal toast topped with grilled tomatoes and ¹/₂oz (12g) grated Edam cheese, 5 fl oz (125ml) unsweetened fruit juice
- ¹/₂ grapefruit or slice of melon, 1¹/₂oz (38g) unsweetened cereal with milk from allowance, 2 crispbreads with 1 tsp marmalade
- 2 rashers well-grilled streaky bacon, grilled tomatoes, mushrooms poached in water, 1 slice wholemeal toast with a little low-fat spread, 1 satsuma
- 1 size 3 egg, boiled, slice of wholemeal toast, 1 apple
- 1 Shape yogurt, 1 slice wholemeal bread topped with 1 tsp peanut butter, 1 pear
- Sandwich of 2 slices wholemeal bread, tomatoes, 1 well-grilled low-fat chipolata, chopped

LUNCHES (choose *one*)

- 1 medium bap spread with mild mustard, 1oz (25g) lean ham, salad with Basic Salad Dressing, 1 large banana, Digestive biscuit
- Sandwich of 2 slices wholemeal bread, 1¹/₂oz (38g) grated Edam cheese with 1 tsp tomato ketchup, 1 orange

- Crusty wholemeal roll with 2oz (50g) chopped cooked chicken, 1 packet low-fat crisps, a few grapes
- 1 McDonald's cheeseburger, 1 apple
- 1 pot Golden Wonder Pot Noodles
- 2 slices wholemeal toast with grilled tomatoes, 1 size 3 poached egg, 1 small banana
- 1 can Weight Watchers from Heinz slimmers' soup, 1 crusty roll, 3oz (75g) chicken breast with huge salad or vegetables from 'free' list
- 10oz (250g) jacket potato with one of the following toppings: 1oz (25g) diced lean ham or chicken, 2 heaped tbsp baked beans, 4oz (100g) cottage cheese with pineapple. Followed by 1 apple, pear or orange

Please pile on the 'free' vegetables.

SUPPERS (choose *one*)

Home-cooked meals

- Pork Paprika with 3oz (75g) potato mashed with milk from allowance, a few grapes
- Fatfield Shepherd's Pie, 4oz (100g) peas, 4oz (100g) carrots, Shape Fromage Frais
- 4oz (100g) lean grilled lamb chop, thin gravy, 1 tsp mint sauce, 3oz (75g) boiled potato, 2oz (50g) sweetcorn, 1oz (25g) scoop vanilla icecream
- 6oz (150g) any white fish, grilled with lemon juice and sliced tomatoes, Leeks with Piquant Yogurt Sauce, 1 crusty wholemeal roll with a little low-fat spread and $^{1}/_{2}$oz (12g) Edam cheese
- 3oz (75g) hot or cold roast meat, fat removed, 7oz (175g) jacket potato with small knob low-fat spread, 4oz (100g) peas, 1 frozen mousse

- 4oz (100g) (dry weight) pasta, boiled until cooked but still firm to the touch, tossed in mixture of 1 beaten egg and 2 tbsp fromage frais with 2oz (50g) grated Edam cheese on top, 1 apple
- 4 grilled fish fingers, 4oz (100g) oven chips, 4oz (100g) peas, 1 apple, 1 orange

Pub Choices
- Ham, chicken or tuna salad, no dressing, slice of French bread, no butter, 1 apple
- Small piece of quiche with salad or vegetables from 'free' list, no dressing, small helping icecream

Ready Meals and Takeaways
- Any Findus Lean Cuisine Meal with 8oz (200g) jacket potato and 1 apple or orange to follow
- Any Bird's Eye Menu Master Healthy Options meal, with 'free' salad and vegetables only
- 5in Deep Pan Pizza, with 1 large banana to follow
- 9 McDonald's Chicken McNuggets, with 1 apple or orange to follow
- Tandoori Chicken, with plain boiled rice and 1 apple or orange to follow

TREATS (choose *two* each day)
- 1 apple and 1 small banana
- 1 Diet Ski yogurt and 1 orange
- 1 crusty roll with salad filling
- 1oz (25g) Edam cheese and 1 crispbread

ALCOHOL ALLOWANCE
You may have 1 pint beer, lager or stout or 2 glasses dry wine or 2 short drink 'doubles' with a low-calorie mixer. But do try to have several drink-free nights each week.

LAZY COOKS' PLAN

This is a brilliant plan for men or women who want a diet with the minimum of fuss and bother. All you need to do is to stock up with meals from your local supermarket, and you are off! While you slim, you'll have loads of time for outside activities, so it is a good idea to join a gym or health club or practise the exercises in Chapter Eight.

EVERY DAY $^1/_2$ pint (275ml) skimmed milk for your tea or coffee, unlimited water and mineral water, but go easy on the diet soft drinks. It is particularly vital to vary your meal choices on this diet, otherwise you will get stuck in a boring rut.

FREE VEGETABLES   Choose them from the list on page 35. Frozen vegetables are just as nutritious as fresh, so don't feel guilty about using them to save time. But do buy fresh salads; it is so quick to wash them and serve them up to add bulk and taste to your meal.

MEN   Add 2 extra slices wholemeal bread, and 1 8oz (200g) jacket potato or 3oz (75g) oven chips each day.

CALORIES   About 1200 daily for women, 1500 for men.

BREAKFASTS

- Buy a Kellogg's Cereal Variety pack and have one pack every day with milk from your allowance, plus 5 fl oz (125ml) unsweetened fruit juice and 1 slice toast with a little low-fat spread

LUNCHES (choose *one*)

- 1 can Campbell's Main Course Soup, any flavour, 1 small crusty roll with a little low-fat spread
- Sandwich of 2 slices wholemeal bread with a little low-fat spread and 4oz (100g) cottage cheese
- 1 takeaway jacket potato with baked beans, cottage cheese or Mexican Bean filling, a few grapes
- 1 mug Batchelors Slim a Soup, 1 beefburger in a bun (no onions)
- Sandwich of 2 slices wholemeal bread with chopped hard-boiled egg and 1 tbsp low-calorie salad cream
- Any Boots Shapers pot meal with 1 large banana to follow
- 1 slice wholemeal toast topped with small can (6oz/150g) ravioli in tomato sauce, 1 satsuma

SUPPERS (choose *one*)

- 1 Ross Stir Fry meal, 1 slice bread with a little low-fat spread
- 1 McCain Deep 'n Delicious Pizza or 1 Findus French Bread Pizza, 1 apple or pear
- 1 large slice of melon, 1 Bird's Eye Menu Master Beef Curry with Rice or Chilli con Carne with Rice, Chambourcy Orange and Lemon Mousse
- 1 well-grilled beefburger, 3oz (75g) McCain Oven Chips, 2oz (50g) peas, 1 small chopped banana and apple, served as fruit salad topped with a few grapes
- 3oz (75g) lean roast meat, thin gravy, 2oz (50g) chunk roast potato, 2oz (50g) carrots, 1 Ross frozen mousse
- Any Findus Lean Cuisine ready meal with 3oz (75g) mashed potato made with skimmed milk from allowance

- Bird's Eye Menu Master Healthy Options Seafood Tagliatelli or Vegetable Lasagne, with 1 apple or orange to follow

Please do not forget your 'free' vegetables and salads.

TREATS AND ALCOHOL ALLOWANCE (choose *one* each day)
- 1 glass dry wine
- $^1/_2$ pint beer or lager
- 1 apple and $^1/_2$oz (12g) Edam cheese
- 1 Diet Ski yogurt with 2 Rich Tea finger biscuits
- 2oz (50g) vanilla icecream

VEGETARIAN PLAN

This is a delicious diet for men and women. Even if you are not a vegetarian, it is well worth trying out for the taste and novelty. You will find all the recipes in Part Two.

One or two of our Fatfield slimmers were vegetarians, and several were 'semi-veggies', who ate white meat and fish occasionally but no red meat at all. If you wish, you could swap any of the suppers given for a simple meal of a 10oz (250g) roast chicken leg, barbecue sauce, an 8oz (200g) jacket potato, some fruit and plenty of 'free' vegetables.

The diet is not suitable for Vegans, as it does include some dairy products.

EVERY DAY $^1/_2$ pint (275ml) skimmed milk for your tea and coffee, unlimited water and mineral water. Use artificial sweeteners only.

FREE VEGETABLES   These are obviously very useful for you, and I give one or two ideas on how you can use them imaginatively in the diet. Pile them on, not forgetting the Fatfield principle – eat more, weigh less!

MEN   You may have 2 extra slices of wholemeal bread each day, plus one extra 'treat'.

CALORIES   About 1200 for women, 1500 for men.

BREAKFASTS (choose *one*)

- 1oz (25g) any unsweetened cereal with milk from allowance, 1 slice wholemeal toast with 1 tsp marmalade, 1 small banana
- 2 slices wholemeal toast topped with grilled tomatoes and 1 size 3 poached egg.
- 1 Weetabix with milk from allowance, 1 slice wholemeal toast topped with 2 tbsp baked beans and grilled tomatoes
- Large bowl of fruit salad made by chopping 1 large banana, 1 apple, 1 pear, and topping with a few grapes and 1 small carton low-fat yogurt
- 1 Shredded Wheat topped with 1 chopped apple, a few raisins, and milk from allowance, 5 fl oz (125ml) unsweetened fruit juice

LUNCHES (choose *one*)

- 2 crusty wholemeal rolls, 4oz (100g) tub of Shape Pineapple Cottage Cheese
- Greek Vegetable Soup, 1 crusty wholemeal roll with a little low-fat spread, 1oz (25g) Edam cheese, a few grapes
- 10oz (250g) jacket potato with Barbecue Sauce, 2 crispbreads with a little low-fat spread and $^1/_2$oz (12g) Edam cheese, 1 apple

- Sandwich of 2 slices wholemeal bread, mashed banana and 1 tbsp curd cheese
- Sandwich of 2 slices wholemeal bread, 1 tbsp baked beans, salad from 'free' list, and 1 packet low-fat crisps
- Citrus Salad in Yogurt Dressing, 1 grilled Vegetable Burger (e.g. Dale Pak or Sainsbury's), 1oz (25g) vanilla icecream with 2 wafers
- 1 piece pitta bread, split and filled with 'free' salad and 4oz (100g) carton Shape coleslaw with 1oz (25g) chopped nuts

SUPPERS (choose *one*)
- Cauliflower cheese – have as much cauliflower as you like, with a sauce made from 1oz (25g) Edam cheese, 1 oz (25g) low-fat spread, 1 tbsp flour and $^1/_2$ pint (275ml) skimmed milk. Serve with grilled tomatoes, 2oz (50g) peas, 1 Diet Ski yogurt to follow
- Curry Creole, 2oz (50g) (dry weight) rice, 1 apple
- Aubergine Casserole, 5oz (125g) jacket potato, 1 medium banana
- 3oz (75g) (dry weight) wholewheat pasta with the Tomato Sauce on page 36, 1 crusty wholemeal roll, $^1/_2$oz (12g) grated low-fat cheese, fresh fruit salad of 1 apple, 1 pear, 1 satsuma and a few grapes
- 1 large slice of melon, Braised Leeks, 2oz (50g) (dry weight) brown rice, 2 rings pineapple canned in juice
- St Michael Fresh Vegetable Canneloni or Casserole, 1 crispy roll
- 7oz (175g) jacket potato with topping of 1 5oz (125g) can baked beans, 4oz (100g) carton St Ivel Shape Garlic and Herb Coleslaw

- 4oz (100g) (dry weight) pasta, preferably wholewheat, boiled until cooked but still firm to the touch, tossed in mixture of 1 beaten egg and 2 tbsp fromage frais with 1oz (25g) grated Edam cheese on top, 1 apple
- Sharwood's Mild Vegetable Curry (14.2oz/405g pack), 1 frozen mousse
- 1 Vegetable Burger (e.g Dale Pak or Sainsbury's), the Tomato Sauce on page 36, 3oz (75g) oven chips, 4oz (100g) carrots, 1 large banana

TREATS AND ALCOHOL ALLOWANCE (choose *one* each day)

- 1 glass dry wine
- $^1/_2$ pint beer, lager or stout
- 1 Mars or Snickers fun size bar
- 2 After Eight Mints
- 1 crusty roll with salad from 'free' list

FOUR 'FREE' VEGETABLE IDEAS
As well as serving your 'free' vegetables cooked simply, or as salads, you can also dish them up like this:

1. *As a casserole* Peel and par-cook a selection of vegetables, pile into a casserole and top with tinned tomatoes, herbs, garlic. Cook in the oven until tender and serve with any of the meals above.

2. *As soup* Use a vegetable stock cube (or make your own) as a base, and add chopped, cooked or leftover vegetables. Purée to make a delicious soup to serve, garnished with watercress or parsley, before your meal. Eat as much as you like. Good vegetable combinations are:

leek, celery and watercress; carrot and tomato; cauli-flower and cucumber.

3. *As crudités* Wash and slice a selection of vegetables and serve before your main course with a non-calorie dip of lemon juice, vinegar, crushed tinned tomatoes, garlic and herbs.

4. *As a stir-fry* Use a non-stick pan and cook through the watery vegetables first (sliced tomatoes, cucumber, beansprouts), gradually adding the others so you make a filling stir-fry without adding oil.

SHIFT-WORKERS' PLAN

When you work unusual hours, it can be very difficult indeed to stick to a low-calorie diet. You may be having your 'breakfast' at lunchtime and your 'lunch' in the middle of the night. Change-over days from one shift to another can leave you even more confused, perhaps eating two dinners in one day.

The one big rule to keep at the very forefront of your mind is that you need a good meal *before* you go to work, whether your job is in a hospital, factory, supermarket or office. This is because you need to make sure that you are at your best while you are working. You will therefore be less likely to reach for a snack when energy levels start to flag.

If possible do take packed snacks to work with you while you slim. Even if the canteen is good, you may still be tempted to eat the wrong things.

This version of the Fatfield Diet is deliberately very flexible. On rest days and weekends, you should follow a normal eating pattern with four meals daily. On working days, choose meals with the correct calorie values from the lists given. You are also allowed a 100-calorie treat every day, including alcohol.

EVERY DAY $^1/_2$ pint (275ml) skimmed milk for your tea and coffee, unlimited water and mineral water. Use artificial sweeteners only.

FREE VEGETABLES Choose from the list on page 35. Pack LOTS of vegetables and salads in your 'goodies' box, together with your snacks, and take them to work.

MEN Add 2 slices wholemeal bread or 2 medium rolls, with a little low-fat spread daily, plus 2 extra Treats.

CALORIES About 1250 calories daily for women, 1650 for men (I would *not* advise shift-workers to try to slim on fewer calories than this).

REST DAYS AND WEEKENDS:
- Breakfast: 200 calorie meal
- Lunch: 300 calorie meal
- Dinner: 400 calorie meal
- Any time: 50 calorie snack and 100 calorie treat

NIGHT SHIFTS
First Night of Shift
- Breakfast (10–11am): 200 calorie meal
- Lunch (3–4pm): 300 calorie meal
- Dinner (about 1 hour before leaving for work): 400 calorie meal
- Supper (mid-shift): 200 calorie meal
- Snack (at home, before bed): 50 calorie snack
- Extra (any time): 100 calorie treat

Subsequent nights
- Breakfast (1pm): 100 calorie meal
- Lunch (4pm): 300 calorie meal
- Dinner (about 1 hour before leaving for work): 400 calorie meal
- Supper (mid-shift): 200 calorie meal
- Snack (at home, before bed): 50 calorie snack
- Extra (any time): 100 calorie treat

LATE SHIFTS
- Breakfast (10am): 200 calorie meal
- Lunch (12.30pm): 200 calorie meal
- Dinner (about 1 hour before leaving for work): 400 calorie meal
- Supper (mid-shift): 300 calorie meal
- Snack (at home, before bed): 50 calorie snack
- Extra (at any time): 100 calorie treat

EARLY SHIFTS
- Breakfast (just before setting off for work – or eat it at work, before you start): 200 calorie meal
- Lunch (mid-shift): 300 calorie meal
- After work: 100 calorie meal
- Dinner (with family): 400 calorie meal
- Supper: 50 calorie snack
- Extra (any time): 100 calorie treat

MEAL LISTS
200 Calorie Meals
- 1oz (25g) unsweetened cereal with milk from allowance, 1 large banana
- Sandwich of 2 small slices wholemeal bread, 2oz (50g) cottage cheese
- 1 size 3 boiled egg, 1 slice wholemeal toast

- 1 Diet Ski or Shape yogurt, any flavour, 1 apple, 2 crispbreads with a little Marmite
- 1 small wholemeal roll, 1 rasher well-grilled back bacon
- Large mixed salad from 'free' list with one of the following: $3^1/_2$oz (99g) tuna canned in brine, chopped apple, lemon juice; 8oz (200g) chicken joint, grilled or roast (skin removed); 3oz (75g) grilled ham steak; 3oz (75g) any lean meat
- 1 mug of Batchelors Slim a Soup, any flavour, medium crusty roll with one of the following: 1oz (25g) grated Edam cheese; 2oz (50g) chicken (no skin); 2oz (50g) lean ham

300 Calorie Meals

- Any Findus Lean Cuisine of 300 calories or less (calorie values are all marked on the package)
- 1 well-grilled low-fat sausage, thin gravy, 3oz (75g) mashed potato, 1 small (5oz/125g) can baked beans
- 4 fish fingers or 6oz (150g) any white fish, grilled, 4oz (100g) peas, 2 tbsp tomato ketchup, 1 crispbread
- 5oz (125g) lean lamb chump chop, grilled, 1 tbsp mint sauce, thin gravy, 4oz (100g) each broad beans and carrots, a few grapes
- Pork Paprika, 1 apple or orange
- Fish Casserole, 1 medium banana
- Fatfield Shepherd's Pie
- 5in Frozen Pizza, 8oz (200g) carton Eden Vale Vinaigrette Coleslaw, 1 crispbread
- 1 slice of wholemeal toast topped with one of the

following: 5oz (125g) can baked beans; 1 size 3 poached egg; 1oz (25g) Cheddar cheese; 2oz (50g) sardines canned in tomato sauce; followed by 1 apple and 1 pear or 1 large banana

Packed meals:

- Sandwich of 2 slices bread with salad from 'free' vegetable list and one of the following fillings: 1oz (25g) grated Cheddar cheese, 2oz (50g) (no skin) cold cooked chicken, 2 oz (50g) lean ham
- Crusty roll with filling of salad, plus any of the above sandwich fillings and 1 apple, orange, pear or small banana
- 1 mug Batchelors Slim a Soup, 8oz (200g) chicken leg (no skin), a few grapes

400 Calorie Meals

Choose any of the 300 calorie meals and add 1 slice bread or a small crusty roll with a little low-fat spread, or choose *one* of these recipe meals:

- 2oz (50g) any cooked, lean meat with Bubble and Squeak
- Piquant Mince with Dishy Dumplings, 1 small wholemeal roll
- Bird's Eye Menu Master Seafood Lasagne or Chilli con Carne with Rice
- 1 portion Kentucky Fried Chicken, 1 portion Coleslaw, 1 portion Barbecue Beans
- Toni's Mackerel and Lemon Pâté, 2 crispbreads, 4oz (100g) any roast meat (no skin), thin gravy

100 Calorie Meals and Treats

- 1oz (25g) any unsweetened cereal with milk from allowance
- 1 Diet Ski yogurt, any flavour, with 1 apple or pear
- 2oz (50g) any lean, cooked meat or small carton cottage cheese with 'free' salad or vegetables
- 1 small slice wholemeal toast topped with grilled tomatoes and $^1/_2$oz (12g) grated Edam cheese
- 1 fun size Mars or Snickers bar
- $^1/_2$ pint beer, lager or stout
- 1 glass dry wine
- 1 double pub-measure 'short' drink with low-calorie mixer

50 Calorie Snacks

- 1 sachet Ovaltine Options
- 1 mug Batchelors Slim a Soup and 2 sticks celery
- 3 large dessert plums
- Selection of chopped raw carrots and dip made from 1 small carton natural yogurt with mustard and lemon juice to taste
- 2 crispbreads with a little Marmite

Do not forget those 'free' vegetables and salads.

THE PLATEAU DIET

Perhaps you've been slimming successfully for some time, but still have some weight which just refuses to budge.

During our Fatfield slim-in for the BBC 'Bazaar' programme, a few of our slimmers got stuck on a slimming 'plateau'. They had lost weight slowly but surely (the best way!) for several months, but suddenly found that no weight-loss registered at our weekly weigh-ins. Although one week at 'stalemate' can easily be explained by fluid changes in the body, when it continues for three or four weeks, something is obviously amiss. We ask all our slimmers to fill in a log of everything they eat each week. This is a good idea for anyone who seriously wants to slim. Even if there is no-one to check your log except you, you will be able to pinpoint any weak spots and also those conveniently forgotten moments when you pinched two glacé cherries off the cake you made for your mother-in-law, or stole a Marmite butty from the baby! Men who fill in their weekly logs are often astonished to find that 50 per cent of their daily calories have been consumed in the pub!

At Fatfield, our slimmers bring their log each week for a talk-through with myself or my assistant, Toni. When we examined the logs of our 'plateau' people carefully, we found that they had not been cheating. So, I devised a special diet to help rev up their sluggish metabolism and encourage their bodies to start 'burning' calories again. Here's how it works:

Week One is a maintenance plan of 1500 calories designed to give the body a 'holiday' from dieting. It is divided up into four meals instead of the usual three, to liven up your system. During this week you should aim to walk briskly for one hour each day.

Week Two is a split-calorie plan which allows 900 calories for three days, then 1200 calories for four days. This helps to 'shock' the system into action. Although it sounds very low in calories, this week's foods are carefully chosen to pack as much bulk in as possible, so you never feel hungry. Exercise this week should be increased to one hour's walking, plus a gentle aerobic activity such as swimming two or three times a week.

The two Weeks are repeated alternately, until the weight starts moving again. Then, one of the other diet plans explained in this chapter can be chosen, according to your weight, sex and lifestyle.

WEEK ONE

CALORIES About 1500 daily for women, 1700 for men and women with more than 3 stone (19kg) to lose.

EVERY DAY You can have ½pt (275ml) skimmed milk for your tea and coffee and unlimited water and mineral water. Use artificial sweeteners only.

FREE VEGETABLES Choose from the list on page 35. Eat as much as you can.

MEN (and women with more than 3 stone (19kg) to lose) You can have 2 extra slices of wholemeal bread daily, with a little low-fat spread.

NOW CHOOSE Each day choose one Breakfast, two Light Meals, one Main Meal and one Treat. (Eat one of the Light Meals at lunchtime, and the other whenever suits you – mid-morning, as a snack when you come home from a hard day's work with your tummy rumbling away or even during the evening when you are watching TV.) Vary your meal choices to give you a super variety of nutrients. This is a 'lenient' week, so you can eat out or have a takeaway!

BREAKFASTS (choose *one* each day)

- 1 poached egg, grilled tomatoes, 1 slice of wholemeal toast, watercress and cucumber

- Blackberry and Apple Sundae
- Fisherman's Breakfast
- ½ grapefruit or slice of melon, 1oz (25g) unsweetened cereal with milk from allowance, 2 crispbreads with 1 teaspoon marmalade
- 2 slices of wholemeal toast topped with grilled tomatoes and 1 rasher grilled streaky bacon, watercress or cucumber slices
- ½ medium melon, sliced across with seeds scooped out. Fill the cavity with 2 tablespoons natural, low-fat yogurt, ½oz (15g) muesli and 1 small banana, sliced
- 1 slice of toast topped with 1 small can (5oz/125g) baked beans, grilled tomatoes

LIGHT MEALS (choose *two* each day)

Don't forget to add huge mixed salads and vegetables from the 'free' list on page 35.

- Tuna Bake, medium banana
- Cheese and Apple Toast, 1 carton Diet Ski or Shape Yogurt, 1 pear
- Courgettes with Haricot Beans or Au Gratin, 3 tablespoons plain boiled rice, 1 small carton Shape Sundae
- Any Lean Cuisine slimmer's meal, plus 1 apple, pear or orange
- Mixed Vegetable Casserole, 10oz (275g) chicken leg (no skin, roasted or grilled), a few grapes
- *Sandwiches* Allow 2 slices of wholemeal bread with filling of salad from the free list (page 35) and one of these:

- 2oz (50g) lean ham or chicken (no skin) with 1 teaspoon sweet pickle
- 4oz (100g) cottage cheese with chives
- 1 large mashed banana with a sprinkling of cinnamon
- 3 orange slices and 1 tablespoon Shape Soft Cheese. Add 1 can (10.4oz/295g) Weight Watchers from Heinz soup

- *Baked potatoes* Allow 1 10oz (275g) potato, scrubbed and baked, with one of these toppings:
  - 1 small carton (5oz/150g) natural, low-fat yogurt with sprinkling of curry powder and lemon juice
  - 2 tablespoons baked beans, sliced tomatoes
  - 1 small carton (5oz/150g) Shape Coleslaw salad
  - 1 small can (8oz/227g) tomatoes with 2oz (50g) chopped prawns or shrimps

- *Cold platter* Salad from 'free' list (page 35) with sliced, hard-boiled egg, 2 tablespoons sweetcorn, 1 carton (4oz/100g) cottage cheese with chives or pineapple, onion rings, orange slices, 2 teaspoons raisins

- *Cereal meals* Choose from the following:
  - 2 Weetabix, milk from allowance, 1 large sliced banana
  - 1oz (25g) unsweetened muesli, milk from allowance, 1 Diet Ski yogurt, any flavour, 1 slice of wholemeal toast with 1 teaspoon marmalade
  - 1oz (25g) porridge oats, made up with water, milk from allowance, 1 slice of wholemeal toast topped with sliced tomatoes, 1 Shape Sundae, any flavour

MAIN MEALS (choose *one* each day)

Don't forget your 'free' vegetables (page 35).

Home Cooked

- Bangers and Mash with Onion, Mushroom and Tomato Gravy, 3oz (75g) peas
- Beef Stew with Newcastle Brown Ale, 5oz (150g) baked potato, 1 medium banana
- Spaghetti Bolognese
- 3oz (75g) roast, lean meat, 3oz (75g) dry roast potatoes (par-boil, brush lightly with vegetable oil and brown under the grill), Slimmers' Apple Bread Pudding
- 6oz (175g) any white fish, grilled with lemon juice and sliced tomatoes, 8oz (225g) baked potato, baked apple
- 1 well-grilled beefburger or vegeburger, 3oz (75g) oven chips, 1 small can (7.6oz/215g) spaghetti-in-tomato sauce, grilled tomatoes, 1 small scoop vanilla icecream

Ready Meals and Takeaways

- Any Findus Lean Cuisine meal with 8oz (225g) baked potato and 1 apple or orange to follow
- Tandoori Chicken, 3 tablespoons plain boiled rice and 1 small banana to follow
- Ross Stir Fry Chinese Chicken or Mexican Beef Chilli with 3 tablespoons plain boiled rice and 1 apple, orange or pear to follow
- Any Sainsbury's Healthy Cuisine Meal except Chicken Madras with Turmeric Rice and 1 apple, orange or pear to follow
- Haddock in Batter from chippie, with unlimited vegetables and salad only

Restaurants

- Carvery: Melon cocktail, roast chicken and unlimited vegetables
- Chinese: Prawn Chop Suey and 2 tablespoons plain boiled rice
- Indian: Chicken Tikka, 2 tablespoons plain boiled rice, 1 poppadum
- Steak House: 6oz (175g) fillet or rump steak, 1 small baked potato with no topping

TREATS (choose *one* each day)

- 1 glass of dry wine
- 2 'short' drinks (pub measure) with low-calorie mixers only
- ½pt (275ml) beer or lager (not strong lager)
- 1 fun size Mars or Snickers bar
- 1 small digestive biscuit

WEEK TWO

CALORIES Three days at 900 calories, four days at 1200 calories. (1100 and 1400 calories for men or women with more than 3 stone/19kg to lose).

EVERY DAY ½pt (275ml) skimmed milk for your tea and coffee, unlimited water and mineral water. Use artificial sweeteners only.

FREE VEGETABLES Choose from the list on page 35. Eat as much as you can.

MEN (and women with more than 3 stone/19kg to lose) Add 2 slices of wholemeal bread, ½pt (275ml) beer or lager or 1 glass dry wine.

NOW CHOOSE Each day choose one Breakfast, one Light Meal, one Main Meal and one Treat.

BREAKFASTS (choose *one* each day)

- 1 small glass unsweetened orange juice, 1 slice of wholemeal toast with Marmite, 1 apple

- 1 small wholemeal roll with 1 rasher grilled back bacon and grilled tomatoes

- 1 small carton (5oz/150g) natural, low-fat yogurt whizzed in the blender with 1 tablespoon wheatgerm, 1 large banana

- 2 crispbreads, grilled tomatoes, 2oz (50g) mushrooms poached in water, 1 poached egg, watercress

- ½ grapefruit, grilled with a pinch of cinnamon on top, 1 slice of wholemeal toast with 1 teaspoon honey, 1 Diet Ski yogurt, any flavour

- 1oz (25g) any unsweetened cereal, milk from allowance, sliced apple, small glass unsweetened tomato or pineapple juice

FIRST THREE DAYS

It is very important to eat plenty of your 'free' vegetables (page 35). Make sure you always sit down to a huge plateful of food at lunchtime and suppertime and don't forget your daily 'treat'.

LIGHT MEALS (choose *one* each day)

Quick, cold meals

- 1 crispy roll with filling of salad and one of these:

- 1oz (25g) grated Edam cheese, sliced tomatoes
- 2 tablespoons cottage cheese mixed with 1 teaspoon sweet pickle
- 2oz (50g) lean ham or chicken (no skin)
- Chopped hard-boiled egg mixed with 1 dessertspoon natural, low-fat yogurt and a pinch of curry powder.

Follow with 1 apple, orange, pear, small banana, or 2 medium plums or 10 grapes

- Lemon dip with Fruit Crudités, $^1/_2$ packet low-fat crisps for dunking
- Pasta Salad, crusty wholemeal roll

Soup meals

- 1 can (10.4oz/295g) Weight Watchers from Heinz soup, any flavour, with crusty roll (fill with salad from 'free' list), 1 Harvest Crunch Bar
- Chilled Gazpacho, 1 slice of wholemeal bread or toast, 1 carton Shape Coleslaw
- 1 can Heinz Big Soup, any flavour, 2 crispbreads
- 1 can Sainsbury's Gourmet Crab Bisque, 1 slice of wholemeal bread or toast

Cooked Meals

- Cheesey Fish Snack, Diet Ski yogurt, any flavour
- Cheese and Vegetable Stir Fry, 1 large banana
- Braised Red Cabbage with Apple Cheese, 1 apple, orange or small banana

MAIN MEALS (choose *one* each day)

- 1 5oz (150g) lean lamb chop, grilled, 3oz (75g) mashed potato (made with skimmed milk from allowance), thin gravy

- Large slice melon or ½ grapefruit, any Lean Cuisine Meal (don't forget the huge portion of 'free' vegetables and salad)

- Well-grilled beefburger, 2 tablespoons baked beans, grilled tomatoes, 2oz (50g) mushrooms poached in water, 1 rasher well-grilled streaky bacon, 2 crispbreads

- 8oz (225g) chicken joint, roast or grilled with skin removed, 2 tablespoons sweetcorn or peas, 1 small crusty wholemeal roll

- Onions Stuffed with Baked Beans, 3 tablespoons plain boiled rice, a few grapes

- Pork Chop with Rosemary and Orange Sauce, 1 tablespoon sweetcorn or peas

- Baked Stuffed Aubergine, 3 tablespoons plain boiled rice, 1 scoop vanilla icecream with sauce made from 1 teaspoon jam and hot water

- 6oz (175g) any white fish, grilled with tomatoes, onions, 5oz (150g) baked potato topped with 2 tablespoons natural, low-fat yogurt

TREATS (choose *one* each day)

- 1 Jaffa Cake
- 2 Rich Tea fingers
- Half packet of Polos or Polo Fruits

NEXT FOUR DAYS
LIGHT MEALS (choose *one* each day)
Quick, Cold Meals
- Chicken and Vegetable Salad, 1 Diet Ski yogurt and a few grapes
- Sandwich of two slices of wholemeal bread *or* two small crispy rolls with salad and one of these fillings:
  - 2 sardines, drained and mashed with lemon juice, 1 tablespoon natural, low-fat yogurt, diced cucumber, red and green peppers
  - 1 pear cored and sliced, lemon juice, 1oz (25g) chopped lean ham
  - 1oz (25g) grated Edam with 1 teaspoon sweet pickle

  Add 1 apple, orange, pear or small banana.

Soup Meals
- Any Cross and Blackwell Chunky Soup with 1 small wholemeal roll
- St Michael Cream of Chicken, Chunky Beef and Vegetable or Lentil and Bacon Soup with 2 crispbreads
- Homemade soup: use 1 large can (14oz/397g) tomatoes, 1oz (25g) leftover cold chicken or lean ham, chopped vegetables from 'free' list and 1 tablespoon peas. Cook until the vegetables are tender and serve with 1 crusty wholemeal roll and follow with an apple, orange, pear or small banana

Baked Potato Meals
- Cook 1 10oz (275g) baked potato, and top with one of the following (don't forget that 'free' salad):
- 2 tablespoons natural, low-fat yogurt and ½oz (15g) grated Edam cheese

- 2 tablespoons baked beans and chopped tomato
- 4 tablespoons cottage cheese with chives

Cooked Meals

- Well-grilled beefburger, grilled tomatoes, 2oz (50g) mushrooms poached in water, 1 small can (7.6oz/215g) spaghetti-in-tomato sauce, 1 apple
- 1 slice of wholemeal toast topped with 1 small can (8oz/225g) baked beans, ½oz (15g) grated Edam cheese
- Poached egg on 1 slice of wholemeal toast, grilled tomatoes, large banana

MAIN MEALS (choose *one* each day)

- Any of the meals for First Three Days, with the addition of 1 crusty roll, 1 slice of wholemeal bread or 2 tablespoons plain boiled rice. Or, choose one of the following:
- Liver, Chipolata and Bean Casserole, 2 tablespoons peas, 5oz (150g) baked potato
- Gammon Steaks with Pineapple and Mustard Sauce, 3oz (75g) mashed potato (use skimmed milk from allowance for mashing), 2 tablespoons sweetcorn, 1 Diet Ski yogurt, any flavour
- Any Findus Lean Cuisine ready-meal, with 2 pieces of fresh fruit (apple, orange, pear, small banana, 2 plums or 1 large slice of melon) to follow
- 3oz (75g) any cooked, lean meat or 6oz (175g) any grilled white fish with 3oz (75g) mashed potato (use skimmed milk from allowance), 2 tablespoons peas, thin gravy (for meat only, make it with a stock cube), with a frozen mousse to follow

Eating Out

Try to avoid it this week (you've got next week to look forward to!), but if you must eat out choose one of these:

- Indian: Tandoori chicken, 2 tablespoons plain boiled rice
- Chinese: Prawn chop suey, 2 tablespoons plain boiled rice
- McDonald's: Cheeseburger, small orange juice
- Carvery: Melon, roast chicken and vegetables, fruit sorbet

TREATS (choose *two* each day)

- ½pt (275ml) beer or lager
- 1 glass of dry wine
- 2 'short' drinks (pub measure) with low-calorie mixers only
- 1 fun size Mars or Snickers bar
- 1 carton Diet Ski yogurt, any flavour
- 1 piece fresh fruit
- 1 individual meringue nest topped with ½ tablespoon low-fat fromage frais and 2oz (50g) strawberries or raspberries

THE CURRY DIET

From time to time, the Fatfield slimmers ask me to provide a short-term diet that caters for a specific food passion! I am happy to do this, provided that the diet follows the basic eat-more-weigh-less principle of the plan and provided it is a short-term diet which doesn't allow the slimmer to fall into the trap of eating the same foods all the time. That, as every Fatfield slimmer knows by now, is bad for your health as well as unlikely to help you slim. A varied diet will provide more nutrients than a boring one! You'll also be less likely to give up!

This 1250/1500 calorie programme was originally devised for a husband and wife slimming team who wanted to lose a few pounds each before going on holiday. Like an increasing number of people, they just love eating curry, and they felt that their waistlines were expanding because of this habit.

It's easy to see why curry lovers put on weight. Normally, people eat a curry as a late-night extra. So, unless they starve all day (which is not a good idea) that day's calorie intake is increased by an enormous amount. Then, after a big blow-out, they go to bed on a very full tummy, which is the quickest way to put on weight.

So, where do the extra calories come from? Well, an average portion of Meat Madras (540 calories), with a couple of chapatis (140 calories each), some pilau rice (470 calories) and 2 tablespoons of mango chutney (80 calories each) add up to 1450 calories. That's enough for a whole day's meals!

On the Fatfield Curry Diet, you can still eat out at Indian restaurants, or you can prepare your own spicy meals at home. The supermarkets now stock so many curry-flavoured ready-meals, canned vegetables and ingredients that it is simple to whip up tasty Indian-style dishes.

EVERY DAY You may have ½pt (275ml) skimmed milk for your tea and coffee and unlimited water (drink lots!). Use artificial sweeteners only.

MEN (and women with more than 3 stone/19kg to lose) You can have 2 extra poppadums or 1 chapati, plus ½pt (275ml) of lager every day!

FREE VEGETABLES Choose them from the list on page 35. Eat plenty. If you like, spice up salads with a dash of paprika or other spices in the Fatfield Dressings. You can also add spices and curry powder to 'free' vegetables like canned tomatoes, courgettes, green beans or cauli- flower to make a basic vegetable curry that is *free*. Eat as much as you like.

CALORIES About 1250 daily for women, 1500 for men and women with more than 3 stone (19kg) to lose.

NOW CHOOSE Each day choose one Breakfast, one Lunch, one Supper and one Treat. NB: All rice is the plain boiled type.

BREAKFASTS (choose *one* each day)

- ½ can (8oz/225g) Heinz Curried Beans with Sultanas, 1 slice of wholemeal toast, 1 small apple
- 5fl oz (150ml) unsweetened orange juice, 1 large slice of wholemeal toast with a little low-fat spread and 2 teas- poons ginger preserve
- 1oz (25g) porridge made with water, milk from allow- ance, 1 small carton (5oz/150g) natural, low-fat yogurt with 2 teaspoons mango chutney stirred in
- 1 egg, boiled and shelled, topped with sauce made from ½ large can (14oz/397g) tomatoes, 1 teaspoon curry powder with 1 slice of wholemeal toast

LUNCHES (choose *one* each day)

- 1 can (6½oz/185g) John West Tuna in Curry sauce, large mixed salad, 1 poppadum
- 1 can St Michael Vegetable Curry, 2oz (50g) cold chicken (no skin), 1 banana

- Curry sandwich: 2 slices of wholemeal bread spread with 3oz (75g) cottage cheese, a pinch of curry powder and sliced cucumber, 1 small carton natural, low-fat yogurt with 1 dessertspoon mango chutney stirred in
- Takeaway: 1 portion Tandoori chicken, huge mixed salad with lemon dressing, a few grapes
- 1 pot Golden Wonder Chicken Curry Meal, cucumber and tomato salad, 1 apple, 2 crispbreads
- 1 Sainsbury's Onion Bhagia with ½ can (16oz/425g) Sainsbury's Chilli beans in Chilli sauce, huge mixed salad

SUPPERS (choose *one* each day)

At home

- Findus Chicken Korma Ready Meal, large mixed salad and cucumber raita (mix 2 tablespoons natural, low-fat yogurt with cucumber slices and lemon juice to taste) (*See* also recipe in Chapter Fourteen)
- Tesco Chicken Vindaloo with Pilau Rice, large green salad, a few grapes
- Sainsbury Vegetable Dhansak, 2 tablespoons plain boiled rice, 1 apple or orange
- Ross Indian Chicken Stir-Fry, 2 tablespoons plain boiled rice, large mixed salad with lemon juice dressing, 1 pear
- Quick Keema, 2 tablespoons plain boiled rice, sliced apple, cucumber and celery salad with lemon juice and sprinkling of chilli powder, 1 banana baked with pinch of ginger
- Fruity Quorn Curry, 4 tablespoons plain boiled rice, 1 small carton (5oz/150g) natural, low-fat yogurt with sliced cucumber and lemon juice

- 1 10oz (275g) chicken leg (skin removed), grilled or roast with sauce made from large portion 'free' vegetables flavoured with spices and curry powder to taste, 6oz (175g) baked potato
- 6oz (175g) any white fish, baked or grilled with sliced tomatoes, onion, lemon juice and paprika, 1 small can (8oz/225g) Heinz Curried Beans, vegetables and salad from 'free' list (page 35)

At the curry house

- Chicken tikka (as Main Course), 2 tablespoons pilau rice, 2 tablespoons cucumber raita
- Tandoori chicken, green salad, 1 chapati
- Mixed vegetable curry, green salad

TREATS (choose *one* each day)

- 1 glass of dry wine
- ½pt (275ml) beer or lager (or save it up for Friday night)
- 1 pack KP Poppadums
- 1 poppadum with 2 tablespoons natural, low-fat yogurt and dash of curry powder for dunking

THE COUPLES' DIET

The Fatfield Diet is fine for whole families, because the meals are so filling. All you have to do is add extra helpings of the more calorie-intensive foods like meat and cheese for non-slimmers. You will probably end up eating bigger platefuls than they do because you'll have unlimited vegetables from your 'free' list (page 35).

If you have a partner who is as anxious to lose weight as you are, it is a good idea to slim together. Then, you can encourage each other all the way. This diet was created for couples who enjoy delicious food, but haven't a lot of time to prepare it. The suppers (or lunches, see below) are slightly higher in calories than usual to allow for man-sized appetites and to make your main meal together special.

While you're following the diet, take up a sport or go to exercise classes together. If either of you is very over-weight, he or she should check with their doctor before embarking on a fitness programme. Give your partner an incentive with a gift or outing for every 7lb (3kg) lost. Keep an eye on each other at parties or when you are both out with friends. Have a special code – a pinch, tickle or wink – which means 'Stop, you're eating, or drinking too much!'.

The diet can also be followed by a lone slimmer, but do invite a friend around to share some of the delicious lunches and suppers!

EVERY DAY You can have ½pt (275ml) skimmed milk for your tea and coffee, and unlimited water. Use artificial sweeteners only.

FREE VEGETABLES Choose from the list on page 35. Don't forget to stock up with frozen vegetables in case you are both too busy to go to the shops or market. Remember that it is great fun to shop together, and less tiring than trying to do it alone. My husband Patrick and I are both dedicated slimmers. We do our bulk shopping every fortnight, and reward ourselves afterwards with a slap-up, low-calorie meal – often the Moules Marinières dish, with fresh mussels from the local fish stall. We add a huge mixed salad, some crusty bread and still have calories left for a glass of dry white wine each!

MEN Add 2 extra slices of wholemeal bread and ½pt (275ml) beer or lager each day.

CALORIES About 1200 daily for women and 1500 for men (or women with more than 3 stone/19kg to lose).

NOW CHOOSE Each day choose one Breakfast, one Lunch, one Supper and one Treat. You may swap around the Lunch and Supper meals if you normally eat your main meal at lunchtime.

BREAKFASTS (choose *one* each day)

- Large slice melon with ginger, 1 poached egg on toast, grilled tomatoes
- 1oz (25g) any unsweetened cereal, milk from allowance, 1 large banana
- Fruity Breakfast Roll
- 5fl oz (150ml) unsweetened orange juice with 1 glass of dry sparkling wine, 2 crispbreads spread with 1 teaspoon strawberry or raspberry jam
- 2 slices of wholemeal toast topped with 2 tablespoons cottage cheese, and a few grapes
- 1 Weetabix biscuit with milk from allowance, 1 sliced pear, 1 slice of wholemeal toast with 1 teaspoon marmalade

LUNCHES (choose *one* each day)

- Cottage Baked Potato with Minty Tomato Salad
- Sandwich of 2 slices of wholemeal bread with any of the fillings from the Fantastic Fatfield Fillings list in

94

chapter twelve plus 2 pieces of the following fresh fruit: apple, orange, medium slice melon, small banana 2 large plums, 10 grapes, $^1/_2$ mango or 1 nectarine

- 2 medium wholemeal rolls with filling of salad from 'free' list plus two of the following:
  - 1oz (25g) grated low-fat Cheddar cheese with 1 teaspoon sweet pickle
  - 1 sliced apple, lemon juice and 1 tablespoon Shape Soft Cheese
  - 2oz (50g) lean, cooked ham or chicken (skin removed)
- 1 small can slimmer's soup, any flavour, 4oz (100g) any grilled white fish or shellfish, huge mixed salad from 'free' list, 5oz (150g) baked potato
- 2 eggs, beaten with 1 dessertspoon skimmed milk, salt and freshly ground black pepper, cooked as an open omelette in a heavy-based, non-stick pan with just a little oil or butter, with a filling of 4oz (100g) frozen mixed vegetables and $^1/_2$oz (15g) grated Edam cheese
- Gazpacho, 1 crusty wholemeal roll with salad from 'free' list (page 35) and 1oz (25g) Edam cheese or 2oz (50g) cold turkey or chicken (skin removed), 1 apple
- 4oz (100g) cottage cheese mixed with 2oz (50g) peeled prawns, $^1/_4$ cucumber peeled and diced, 2oz (50g) canned asparagus, drained and chopped. Serve, seasoned with freshly ground black pepper on a bed of lettuce leaves, plus 1 5oz (150g) baked potato

SUPPERS (choose *one* each day)
- Lovers' Dinner, 1 glass of dry wine

- 5oz (150g) lean rump steak, 3oz (75g) McCain Oven chips, vegetables and salad from 'free' list (page 35), 1 scoop vanilla icecream with 1 teaspoon jam diluted with 1 tablespoon unsweetened orange juice
- Low Calorie Fish and Chips, $^1/_2$ pt (275ml) lager or glass of dry white wine, huge mixed salad from 'free' list (page 35), a few grapes
- Moules Marinières, 4oz (100g) chicken breast poached in 1 can slimmer's mushroom or chicken soup, vegetables from 'free' list, 3oz (75g) mashed potatoes made with skimmed milk, baked apple
- Hummus, 2 crispbreads, Cheese and Vegetable Stir Fry, 1 crusty wholemeal roll, 1oz (25g) low-fat Cheddar cheese
- 3oz (75g) any lean roast meat, thin gravy, huge pile of vegetables from 'free' list (page 35), 3oz (75g) large chunk or chunks of roast potato (cooked the Fatfield Way, see page 205), 2oz (50g) carrots, Apricot and Yogurt Icecream, or 1 Diet Ski yogurt, any flavour, and 1 apple or orange

TREATS (choose *one* each day)
- 1 glass of dry wine
- ½pt (275ml) beer or lager
- 2 'short' drinks (pub measure) with low-calorie mixers
- 1 fun size Mars or Snickers bar
- Chambourcy Creme Caramel
- Shape Sundae and a few grapes
- Ambrosia Pot Low Fat Rice
- 2 Jaffa Cakes

CHAPTER SIX

HOW OUR SLIMMERS COPED

Here are some inspiring stories from our original group of Fatfield Slimmers. Anyone who has ever been overweight will recognise many of the problems that these super people had before they changed their eating habits. In some cases, the pounds had piled on gradually over the years. In others, there were medical or emotional reasons why they had put on weight.

As the pounds dropped off, it was exciting to see how much healthier and more active everyone became. Toni, my assistant, and I noticed that people seemed busier and busier. People who had been coming along to our regular weigh-ins wearing ordinary clothes, suddenly started turning up in skin-tight leotards and cycling shorts! Not only that, they had fitted in an aquafit or exercise session before our meeting.

The social scene in Fatfield is pretty active anyway, but we found that some slimmers had so much energy they were able to dance the night away, even after a tough day at work.

Vera Churnside joined a car maintenance class, and along with her sister-in-law Julie Mulvaney, took part in a charity fun run. Which all proves that the right diet makes you *feel* terrific as well as *look* tons better!

Name: **Lynn Ayre**
Age: 28 *Occupation*: Full-time mother *Height*: 5ft 10in
Starting weight: 14st 13lb *Weight after 20 weeks*: 11st 10lb

Attractive Lynn Ayre bought a slinky black Lycra dress to celebrate losing 2 stone on the Fatfield Diet . . . and now it is too big for her!

Lynn says, 'I feel like a different person. The old, frumpy me is gone for good. I'm now having more fun than ever before and strangely enough, I am eating *more* than ever.'

She has always been tall and well built (like so many of our Fatfield slimmers), but ten years ago she weighed a reasonable $11^1/_2$ stone.

'But, then I got married,' she says, 'and had my two children, Chris and Vicky. Chris was born in 1984, and I ballooned to 18 stone during the pregnancy. After Vicky was born in 1987, I managed to get down to $12^1/_2$ stone on a semi-starvation diet.'

Then, not surprisingly, Lynn began to put *on* weight. 'I would begin a diet on Monday, and forget it by Tuesday,' she says. 'With two small children to look after, I was snacking all the time instead of eating proper meals. I seemed to live on biscuits and toast and butter.'

Sadly, Lynn's marriage broke up, and she began to eat even more of the wrong foods because she was so depressed. However, in terms of bulk, her daily food intake was not that excessive. For instance, a typical day's breakfast would be cereal, and a couple of slices of toast and butter.

'Then, I'd go shopping and have a pie and some chips. Later, instead of having a proper meal with the children, I would have a takeaway or more snacks. It didn't seem very much, but I now realise that it was all fat-laden. At the time, I just didn't think it was worth cooking something healthy just for me.'

On Fridays and Saturdays, Lynn would enjoy a few half-pints of strong vintage cider at around 200 calories each.

Christmas 1990 was especially difficult for Lynn. 'I weighed over 15 stone, and had to be dragged out to visit friends and relatives. Even though it was the festive season, I spent the whole time dressed in baggy skirts and jumpers or covered my bulges with huge T-shirts. My bust measurement was 44FF.'

Then, Lynn's doctor advised her to lose weight. 'What he had to say made sense. I could see that I was in danger of ruining my health. So, when the Fatfield experiment started in January 1991, I was one of the first to volunteer. But I was so worried that I would be one of the fattest people there that, before I went along to the weigh-in, I actually lost a few pounds by eating very little.'

At first, Lynn did not believe that she would ever be able to eat as much food as was specified on her version of the diet – the Steady Weight Loss Plan.

'I started piling on the vegetables, as instructed, and planning my meals ahead instead of grabbing snacks in a casual way. It was fun, and made me feel so much better about myself.'

Lynn now checks in with her own doctor once a fort-night, follows the diet carefully, and has also joined an aerobics class.

'It seems to be a real turning point in my life,' she says. 'I am thinking much more positively, and have bags more energy. Soon, both my children will be at school, so I hope to get a part-time job, perhaps in a shop. I feel so much more confident about my appearance these days. The other day, I bumped into a couple of friends I haven't seen for five years and they didn't recognise me. It was a great feeling.'

Name: **Pam Orwin**
Age: 27 *Occupation*: Barmaid *Height*: 5ft 8in
Starting weight: 15st 1lb *Weight after 20 weeks*: 12st 7lb

At first, Pam was a reluctant subject for our Fatfield experiment. 'Frankly, I have tried so many diets that I didn't believe that this one would work,' she says. 'In my job, it is very difficult indeed to lose weight. People try to get you to have a drink and even if you don't, you're tempted to eat crisps and bar snacks. When you get home, you're so tired that you grab a sandwich or some biscuits.'

But Pam, who has two small children, wasn't prepared for the change in her looks and the way she felt.

'For the first time, I actually began to enjoy putting on make-up and dressing up. Most people complain when the weight comes off their face but I was delighted. Suddenly, I had high cheekbones! Admittedly, the weight came off my hips and waistline too and I started to try on skirts and tops that I hadn't worn for years.'

'The best part is that I am never hungry.'

Pam has now signed up for a college course in business studies, and is looking forward to returning to work when her children need less attention.

'I could never go back to my old eating habits now,' she says.

Name: **Susan Smith**
Age: 36 *Occupation*: Laboratory technician
Height: 5ft 4¹/₂in
Starting weight: 10st *Weight after 20 weeks*: 8st 9lb

When Susan joined the Fatfield Diet experiment, she was extremely doubtful that she would ever be able to stick to *any* diet, let alone ours. She had a long list of food allergies, including wheat, rye, citrus fruits, and dairy products. She also had a history of asthma, and frequent use of steroids to control it had pushed her into a 'yo-yo' syndrome of gaining and losing weight. Although she only wanted to lose a stone or so, she was fearful that another bout of asthma could knock all her slimming intentions for six.

'I have put on as much as 10lb in a week on steroids,' says Susan. 'I had a very bad bout of asthma just a month before joining the slimming group. It began when my dog died in September 1990, then I had flu and generally went to pot!'

Susan's pretty eleven-year-old daughter Katherine is a keen rider and owns a horse called Angel. Unfortunately, her mother's asthma was triggered by close contact with Angel, and this caused them both a lot of distress. 'On one particularly bad day, I had to just leave Katherine at the stable and dash home because I was in such a state. It was very upsetting for both of us.'

We simply tailored the basic Fatfield Diet to suit Susan, by knocking out foods she cannot eat and drink and, where possible, replacing them with things she can. Ordinary milk was replaced by soya milk; she had melon, plums or nectarines instead of citrus fruits; and porridge oats (she is not allergic to oats) instead of other cereals for breakfast. She also ate oat cakes, feta cheese (which doesn't upset her), and had a packet of low-fat crisps as her daily 'treat'.

She lost weight slowly but surely. On the first weigh-in, about three weeks after we started, we found that she was down to 9st 11lb, then the scales registered 9st 9lb, and so on.

'The most interesting thing was that, as my diet improved, my asthma attacks stopped, and I felt tons healthier,' says Susan. 'I always carry an inhaler, but I haven't had to use it for ages.'

Susan now attends no fewer than *five* fitness classes a week, despite her demanding job as a laboratory assistant. She is doing an Open University BA degree and is determined to learn to ride. In May, she completed a 6 mile fun run for charity, with her inhaler in her hand – but is delighted to report that she didn't have to use it!

Name: **Erika Lowdon**
Age: 63 *Occupation*: Retired Postwoman
Height: 5ft 1in
Starting weight: **10st 3lb** *Weight after 20 weeks*: **8st 7lb**

Erika is a mum-in-a-million who believes that the Fatfield Diet helped her get into fighting form before undergoing major surgery recently. She was born in Germany where she met her husband Austin when he was stationed there during his National Service tour of duty. The couple have three grown-up children and five grandchildren. Erika's story is truly inspirational.

'I retired from my job as the local postwoman in April 1989,' she says. 'After walking between seven and nine miles a day for thirty years of my life, I was suddenly taking far less exercise. Naturally, I began to put on weight.'

Within a short time, she had expanded from around 9 stone to over 10 stone. It was not disastrous, but Erika was very annoyed with herself.

'I didn't want to get fatter and fatter as I got older,' she says. 'Then, at around the same time, I went along for a routine health check and found that I had a slow-developing type of breast cancer. It was a shock, but something that I just had to cope with.'

Eventually, the cancer became worse, and Erika's doctor told her that radical surgery would be necessary.

'I made up my mind to have an implant operation at the same time, which meant surgery on both breasts. And, I also decided to lose the weight I'd put on and get extra fit before the op, scheduled for March 1991!'

With her doctor's permission, Erika joined our group at the end of January 1991, at the same time as her daughter, Maureen.

'As soon as I started the diet, I knew I had made the right decision,' she says. 'The foods are healthy and delicious and fit into our family life. Austin particularly enjoys the Fatfield Shepherd's Pie and a lamb casserole. At weekends, the whole family often come over, and I'll serve up Fatfield-style meals like a chicken stir-fry, or even oven-baked fish and chips. Austin has a wonderful variety of produce on his allotment, so we always have a good choice of "free" vegetables to choose from.'

'My doctor was pleased too, because so many women put *on* weight during the recovery period after this kind of surgery, and he felt that I would get a psychological boost from looking slim while I was getting over the operation.'

Erika found that she enjoyed the diet tremendously, and even joined the Aquafit class with Maureen. She went into hospital feeling positive and optimistic, weighing just under $9^{1}/_{2}$ stone.

After a ten-day stay in hospital, Erika went straight back onto the diet, and weighed in at 9st 1lb three weeks afterwards.

'I'd advise any woman facing this kind of operation to go on a healthy eating plan – it helps you cope with your worries, and makes you feel very positive. I am now looking forward to keeping my weight steady at $8^{1}/_{2}$ stone!'

Name: **Rose Irwin**
Age: 45 *Occupation*: Housewife *Height*: 5ft
Starting weight: **15st 9lb** *Weight after 20 weeks*: **13st 9lb**

Warm, welcoming Rose is a great cook and loves entertaining. But, until she discovered the Fatfield Diet, Rose was using a couple of pounds of lard a week for her famous roast dinners and Yorkshire puddings! Now, she is committed to the fat-free Fatfield style of cuisine, and has lost 2 stone to prove it.

Like so many other women, Rose put on weight when she gave up her job to become a full-time housewife. Now, she looks after her husband and two grown-up sons – who all have healthy appetites.

'I had an arm injury so I had to stop my factory job,' she says. 'I found I had time to make cakes, puddings and filling supper dishes. The family gained a lot . . . and so did I!'

Rose was the first Fatfield slimmer to allow the BBC 'Bazaar' camera crew into her home – while she prepared a superb Sunday lunch. Later, she showed *us* how to make a perfect Fatfield Shepherd's Pie.

'One of the first things I did on the diet was to throw out all my old baking tins and buy new, non-stick ones,' she says. 'It was a great excuse for a spending spree. I hadn't realised that you could make Yorkshire puddings without using lard, or cook chips without a chip pan.'

'I'm one of these women who has clothes in their wardrobes which cover all sizes from 14 to 22,' says Rose. 'But now, I'm convinced that I will soon be throwing out the large-size outfits for good.'

'The weight is coming off steadily, I feel full up all the time, and I have even joined the Aquafit sessions at the local pool.'

Name: **Vera Churnside**
Age: 30   *Occupation*: Housewife   *Height*: 5ft 6^1/$_2$in
Starting weight: 10st 6lb   *Weight after 20 weeks*: 10st

Name: **Russell Churnside**
Age: 32   *Occupation:* Senior Fresh Food Manager
Height: 5ft 6in
Starting weight: 12st 5lb   *Weight after 20 weeks*: 11st 2lb

Vera and Russell are a lively, young couple with three beautiful little daughters and lots of friends. Julie Mulvaney, one of our other Fatfield slimmers, married Vera's brother in June 1991, keeping the whole thing strictly in the family!

A few months before they started the Fatfield Diet, both Vera and Russell felt decidedly unfit.

'Recently, I looked at a picture of myself wearing a favourite bright pink dress, and I just couldn't believe how plump I looked,' says Vera. 'I used to pour myself into jeans, which now fit me perfectly. My waist has shrunk from 30 inches to 26 inches.'

Russell, although not fat, was concerned that he was getting far too hefty for a man of his height and age.

'I was snacking between meals, and eating too many fatty foods,' he says. 'We both felt in need of a fitness boost.'

The results have been truly spectacular. The Churnsides now look like a different couple. Just check out the pictures of them, and you will see what I mean. Their weight-loss has been painless, with *lasting* results. Their super new eating habits have made them feel amazingly energetic too.

Vera, with her 26-inch waistline, looks five years younger than her real age, and says, 'If you had told me six months ago that I would now be going to fitness classes every single day, I would have laughed. But I feel absolutely marvellous!'

Russell admits that he has had the occasional slip-up on the diet. 'In my job, it is very difficult to resist the occasional cream cake, so I don't try. Instead, I have learned how to make up for any indiscretions by being especially good the next day,' he says.

To celebrate his new shape ('He's even more gorgeous-looking than he was before,' says his wife!), Russell has just achieved a lifetime's ambition by going hang-gliding.

Name: **Julie Mulvaney**
Age: 25 *Occupation*: Play Area Assistant in a DIY super-store *Height*: 5ft
Starting weight: **12 st 7lb** *Weight after 20 weeks*: **11st 7lb**

Julie was married at the local Methodist church during the Fatfield slim-in. Despite that incentive, for the first month of the programme she experienced some difficulty in losing weight. We were perplexed, because, on the Fatfield Diet, it is impossible *not* to lose weight if you follow it correctly.

'I admit that I cheated,' says Julie. 'My husband, John, is a long-distance lorry driver and he is sometimes away on the Continent for weeks at a time.'

'Before our wedding, I was often very lonely indeed, sitting for hours in our flat just watching television or trying to read. So, to comfort myself, I ate sweets, chocolates, fish and chips and Chinese takeaways *as well as* the foods listed on the diet.'

Julie was also under a lot of pressure to lose weight for her big day. 'Friends were always nagging me to shape up, and somehow that made everything worse. When I looked in the mirror, I couldn't see how I could possibly look good on my wedding day. It was a nightmare because the worse I felt, the more I wanted to cheat!'

The turning point for Julie came when she came down to London for a 'make-over' session at the famous John Frieda hair salon. Theresa Fairminer, who has made up many famous women, including the Duchess of York, showed Julie how to slim her face with clever make-up, and Ian Denson re-styled her hair.

'When they'd finished, I almost dreaded looking in the mirror,' says Julie. 'But I looked so good, that I realised that I *could* be a slim, beautiful bride after all.'

From that day onwards, Julie had no trouble at all in sticking to her diet . . . and she is still following it faithfully. 'I have a filling Fatfield breakfast of bran cereal and a banana before I go to work, a canteen lunch at work which is usually a huge salad, with yogurt to follow. For supper, I eat one of the meals on the diet plan, or, if I've worked a late night, I make myself a vast sandwich, stuffed with all the "free" vegetables and chicken or tuna. I eat it slowly, and then nibble lots of fruit. As a late night "comfort" drink, I sip a mug of Ovaltine Options, which is delicious and only 40 calories.'

Julie is still losing weight steadily, at the rate of about 2lb a week. Her goal is $8^{1}/_{2}$ stone.

Name: **Janine**
Age: 32   *Occupation*: Dancer   *Height*: 5ft
Starting weight: **9st 8lb**   *Weight after 20 weeks*: **9st 1lb**

Janine is married with a young daughter and leads a hectic life as a dancer. She performs with her own three-girl group, Two Tone, for promotions and in clubs and pubs.

When she came along to the Fatfield weigh-in, she had been trying desperately to lose weight for some time on a crazy diet that consisted of periods of starvation followed by orgies of chocolate biscuits!

It took us some time to convince Janine that she was not eating enough, and was in danger of damaging her health on this mad plan. We were more concerned about helping her to eat healthily and to stabilise her weight than slimming her down! I explained that she would need to eat *more* and that her metabolism would be erratic for some time before we could establish a steady weight-loss pattern.

'Dancers survive on adrenaline, cigarettes and chocolate,' she says. 'I tried to lose a few pounds by cutting out virtually everything. For some time, I lived on around 600–800 calories a day, mostly chocolate.'

On her first week on the Fatfield Diet, Janine put *on* 4lb. This was not surprising as she was taking in around 600 calories more than before. She was disappointed, but felt much fitter and decided to carry on.

She took packed meals with her to the pubs and clubs where she appears, so that she was never 'caught short' without the right food. Wholemeal sandwiches, fruit, and diet soft drinks replaced her usual post-performance snack of a bar of chocolate and a fizzy, sugar-laden drink.

Within two months, Janine's weight stabilised and her body changed shape. 'I noticed that my waist and bottom were getting smaller, and there was less flab on my body,' she says. 'I also felt a whole lot fitter. Before going on the diet, I used to just crash out after a hectic day's work. Now, I go to Aquafit classes, and aerobics as well as practising my own routines. I have bags of energy.'

At the time of writing, Janine has started losing weight steadily and safely. She aims to get down to around $8^1/_2$

stone, which is fine for her height, bearing in mind that a dancer's fat–muscle ratio is different from that of a woman who takes little or no exercise.

Slimmers like Janine who have been on semi-starvation diets can safely use the Fatfield Diet. But, results will be slower, and you could put on a few pounds at first, as Janine did. Stick with it, because you *will* lose weight eventually – and this time it will stay off.

Name: **John Herkes**
Age: 56   *Occupation*: Retired Security Guard
Height: 5ft 10in
Starting weight: **13st 10lb**   *Weight after 20 weeks*: **12st 6lb**

Bang in the middle of his Fatfield slim-in, John gave up smoking. Yet he continued to lose weight steadily.

'I was a regular twenty-a-day smoker until April 1991, about half-way through the Fatfield experiment,' he says. 'I imagined that my weight would go up when I quit, but it didn't. I am delighted with my weight-loss.'

John's wife Ann lost over a stone on the diet and they both feel very fit.

'We used to eat pies, chips, fried bacon, sausages and more chips,' says John. 'Now, we both pile our plates high with vegetables and never feel deprived.'

John's weight-loss pattern was typical of many men on the diet. He lost 13lb in the very first week! But then, the pounds came off more gradually, until he gave up smoking. Even then, we registered a weight-loss of one to two pounds weekly.

Meanwhile, Ann lost a massive half-stone in the first week, then a steady one or two pounds until she reached her goal of $9^{1}/_{2}$ stone.

John maintains that the high-fibre foods were so satisfying that they reduced his craving for cigarettes. I would like to hear from other slimmers who have given up smoking and tried the diet. Please write to me at the address on page 121, and let me know how you got on. For many people, the one thing that puts them *off* giving up the dreaded weed is the prospect of ballooning in weight. This diet could be the answer to this common problem.

Name: **Debbie Herkes**
Age: 27 *Occupation*: Clerical Worker *Height*: 5ft 5in
Starting weight: **9st 13lb** *Weight after 20 weeks*: **9st 4lb**

Debbie, who is the daughter of John and Ann Herkes, started the diet knowing that she faced a two-week holiday in Portugal right in the middle of her slimming campaign.

'I was worried that I would put on loads of weight during the holiday,' she says. 'I started off wrongly by following the local custom of eating late at night. We'd have a fairly large breakfast, a sandwich and drink at lunchtime and then a big meal at around 10pm. I found that I had headaches, felt bloated, and couldn't sleep too well. So, I quickly decided to switch back to eating earlier, at around 7pm. I chose salads and fish dishes, but it was quite difficult to avoid things smothered in oil.'

Pretty Debbie put *on* 5lb during her holiday, but within a week of going back on the Fatfield plan, she had lost 7lb.

'The plan works for me because I don't feel hungry between meals,' she says. 'Before I started it, I'd got into the habit of snacking on crisps, biscuits, and chips. My weight was just going up and up. Now, I never feel the need to nibble.'

She feels happy with her current weight – even though it is higher than two years ago, when she weighed in at 8st

4lb. 'I was doing a lot of Karate, to purple- and white-belt standard, and aerobics, but not eating very much. I didn't feel very well, and I looked too thin.'

'Now, I look good, and I feel it too. I am doing some weight training, but using light weights only so I don't get muscle-bound.'

'I save some of my treats for the evening. For instance, if I get peckish while I'm watching television, I have a piece of crispbread and some soft cheese or some fruit.'

If, like Debbie, you go on holiday in the middle of your slimming campaign, do not worry. Try, as far as possible, to choose Fatfield-style foods – salads without dressing, plain grilled meat and fish, fresh fruit, local bread. Avoid butter, cream, rich sauces, and too much alcohol!

When you get home, wait a couple of days before weighing yourself. If you have put on 7lb or more, you cheated *too* much! Less than 7lb. Go on the Quick Weight Loss version of the diet for one week, then back on your normal programme.

Name: **Brenda Taylor**
Age: 37 *Occupation*: Quality Control Operator
Height: 5ft 2in
Starting weight: **11st 8lb** *Weight after 20 weeks*: **9st 5lb**

Brenda came along to our first Fatfield weigh-in just for fun, and ended up by losing 31lb!

She says, 'I went along with my neighbour, Vera Churnside, just to be part of the television crowd scene. Then, I suddenly found myself queuing up to be weighed. I had meant to lose some weight for ages, so I decided to go along with the experiment.'

Brenda has a five-year-old daughter, and a very busy life. Her husband, Roy, runs his own joinery business.

'Roy is one of those infuriating men who can eat any-thing and never puts on weight,' she says. 'Before I went on the Fatfield Diet, I was eating all the wrong things, simply because I didn't realise how fat I was getting.'

Like so many of our slimmers, Brenda used to start the day on an empty stomach. 'By mid-morning I was rave-nous, so I would have a sandwich and a couple of biscuits. Then, I'd nibble more biscuits while deciding what to have for lunch!'

She usually decided to have a pie or another sandwich and more biscuits. At night, she would cook a big meal for the family, and eat it – together with any leftovers.

Now, she has bran cereal and banana for breakfast with milk from her daily allowance and a piece of fruit. Lunch is a healthy salad with slimmer's soup, and supper is one of the Fatfield recipe meals.

Her job is a four-hour shift – from 3pm to 7pm, or 7pm to 11pm. 'I work my meals around my job, making sure that I never miss one,' she says. 'In the evenings, I'll have an Ovaltine Options drink while I read or watch television.'

'Before, I used to crave nibbles and snacks right through the evening, but now I don't miss them at all. What's more, I feel so fit that I have taken up riding on Sundays, with my daughter and Vera. I'm so glad that my Fatfield neighbour got me involved in the plan – even though it was by accident!'

CHAPTER SEVEN

HOW TO STICK TO YOUR DIET

Is your willpower so wobbly that you fear that you will go *off* your diet within a few days of starting it? If so, you must realise that it is vital to prepare yourself mentally to lose weight. It is not an easy thing to do and I get very angry with those who throw scorn at overweight people, calling them 'greedy' or 'fat slobs'. Frankly, I have met very few greedy fat slobs in my time. Almost every overweight person we have counselled over the years has had a very good reason for putting on the pounds. Maybe they have had children in rapid succession, and found it difficult to shape up between pregnancies, or maybe they have had an illness which has made them unable to take exercise. Very often, there are emotional reasons why both men and women overeat. I cannot accept that emotional food cravings are a purely feminine problem. We have worked with many, many men who eat, and drink, too many of the wrong things because they are suffering from stress, depression, or sexual problems. Fat is a human issue, not just a feminist one.

If you are to win the battle of the bulge, you need four important things: the right diet plan, motivation, imagination, and lots of support. Well, you have definitely found the right diet plan, so now let's look at the other three factors:

MOTIVATION

Do have a long, hard think about the *reason* why you want to lose weight. At our first meeting with the Fatfield slimmers, three main reasons emerged. The first two were pretty general: everyone wanted to improve their health and appearance.

There were men like John Herkes who had already given up smoking, put on a bit of weight, and now wanted to be slim and trim as well as free of his nicotine addiction. Then, there was brave Erika Lowdon, who faced serious surgery and wanted to be in top form to help her recover swiftly. Lovely Rose Irwin (who lost 28lb altogether) vowed that she wanted to look good in hot pants and wear them to church to amaze the vicar!

But most of our slimmers had another, strong, personal reason for wanting to lose weight too: such as pretty Julie Mulvaney who was determined to look amazing on her wedding day (she did!); or Pam Orwin, barmaid at The Riverside pub, who decided to look terrific for her first day back at college where she is studying office management; and bakery manager Russell Churnside who wanted to be fit enough to fulfil a life-time's ambition to go hang-gliding. They all managed to achieve these aims by their own brilliant efforts.

Consider these ten good, medical reasons for losing those excess pounds:

1. *Lengthen your life.* It is sad but true that fat people die younger than slim people. According to data collected by the insurance companies, there is a direct connection between early mortality and excess weight. The odds are shortened if you are what is clinically termed 'obese' – that is around 20 per cent overweight.

2. *Beat heart disease.* The fatter you are, the greater the

risk of dying of a heart attack. Your heart has to work harder pumping blood around your body and the level of cholesterol in your arteries increases. So there is a far greater chance of arteries becoming blocked, and your poor old heart giving up the struggle!

3. *Lower your blood pressure.* High blood pressure increases your chances of having a heart attack or a stroke – both can be fatal. If you lose weight, you stand a very good chance of having normal blood pressure levels, which is more fun than taking tablets all your life and constantly living in fear of serious illness.

4. *Prevent aches and pains.* Joint problems such as arthritis and rheumatism are made much worse if you are overweight. The extra pressure makes your joints work harder and they are therefore more likely to wear out. Imagine carrying a couple of 10lb bags of potatoes everywhere – that is what your poor old hips, knee joints and feet have to put up with even if you are merely 1 stone 6lb overweight.

5. *Breathe more easily.* Do you wheeze, cough, and splutter as you struggle upstairs? Have you given up trying to climb up to the top deck of the bus? Do you catch all the colds going every winter? Maybe your lungs are fed up with trying to function properly surrounded by so much flab.

6. *Avoid diabetes.* One type of diabetes occurs in middle or old age, and is triggered by overweight. Controlling it requires patience, a special diet, tablets, or even regular insulin injections. It has been estimated that thousands of fat people are diabetics without realising it, feeling run down and ill all the time.

7. *Make surgery easier.* However fit you are, there are times when surgery can be necessary. If a surgeon has to cut through layers of fat to do a routine operation, then complications become far more likely. Post-operative care takes much longer and recovery is slowed down.

8. *Reduce the risk of infertility.* If you are fat, you reduce your chances of conceiving a baby easily. Fat people who attend infertility clinics are advised to slim down. In any case, it is always wise to get into good shape, and eat a healthy diet before conception, to ensure that your baby has a perfect start.

9. *Beat digestive complaints.* These can vary in seriousness from indigestion, gassiness and pain – all caused by overloading the stomach – to complaints such as gall bladder disease and gall stones which occur more frequently in overweight people.

10. *Enjoy an active sex life.* A loving sex life is good for your health. While there is no doubt that overweight people can have just as much fun in bed as slim people, it is a fact that you feel better about yourself when you are slim. That means you are less likely to be inhibited about sex and more likely to get your fair share and, even more important, to enjoy it!

Now check out these ten cost-cutting reasons for losing weight:

1. Large-size clothes cost more than normal, off-the-peg styles.

2. Cleaning bills mount up when you are fat because you perspire more, and need to change outfits more often.

3. Life insurance policies are expensive if you are huge and unhealthy.

4. Shoes wear out quickly when they are carrying 15 stone of flab around all day long.

5. Car seats and suspension take a bashing when they come into daily contact with a massive bum!

6. Food bills mount up if you are consuming high-calorie foods like cakes, puddings and sweets. The Fatfield Diet is designed to fit in with a family budget.

7. Household wear-and-tear is maximised when there is a large person in the house, flopping on the sitting-room sofa and bouncing on the bed.

8. It is unfair but true that 'fatties' are less likely to get promotion at work than slim people.

9. Holidays become expensive when you have to fork out extra cash for supersized swimsuits and beachwear.

10. You use a lot more of everyday items like washing powder, body lotion, deodorant and soap. Little things do add up!

Most important of all, think positive. Here are five very personal reasons for losing weight, contributed by the Fatfield slimmers. You probably have some of your own. Make a list for yourself.

1. 'I want to wear hotpants in church and amaze the vicar.' (*Rose Irwin*)

2. 'I want to tackle an army assault course, and do really well!' (*Vera Churnside*)

3. 'I'm going to get a fabulous new slimsize costume to wear in my stage dancing act.' (*Janine*)

4. 'I'm going to look marvellous on my wedding day.'
(*Julie Mulvaney*)

5. 'I'm going to be a wow in a bikini on holiday.' (*Debbie Herkes*)

IMAGINATION

It may be a long, long time since you were slim. So, it is hard to picture yourself looking any other shape than you are right now. But, one of the most helpful things you can do during your slim-in is to imagine yourself slim.

Psychologists have found that mental attitude can make or break your slimming campaign. By having your mind 'tuned in' to your new image, it will help your body to conform to *that* image. If this sounds far-fetched, let me tell you that most slimmers who succeed in losing large amounts of weight are those who have a very clear idea of how they might look and behave as slim people. Sometimes, this 'body-image awareness' does not register straight away, but an event, picture in a magazine, or chance remark from a friend triggers it off, so the slimmer has a sudden realisation of just what he or she might look like once the stones and pounds have dropped off. Once that picture is firmly lodged in the brain, bingo! – the diet starts to work.

A good example of this is our gorgeous Fatfield bride, Julie Mulvaney. Julie, who is a play area assistant, would be the first to admit that she was struggling with her diet. She weighed in at $12^1/_2$ stone, and at the third weigh-in, she still weighed exactly the same. It was very puzzling indeed. She says, 'I could not see myself as a slim person. So, I cheated. My husband is a continental lorry driver and away for long periods, so I consoled myself by eating the wrong things. Then, I would miss out on meals – which goes right against the Fatfield Diet principles and is disastrous for someone like me who works, and eats, with children.' Julie needed a real jolt to imagine herself as a slim person and get her going (*see* page 106).

Here are some 'mind over body' exercises *you* can do to help you tune in to the most powerful slimming aid of all, your brain:

1. Spend 10 minutes each day 'psyching' yourself slim. Lie down on a sofa or couch, close your eyes, and breathe regularly for a few moments. Let your mind wander, with different images flitting in and out of your brain. Now focus on an image of yourself, looking slim and fit, in a familiar situation – perhaps at a party, walking along a favourite beach, or entertaining friends at home. You are feeling good, the atmosphere is happy, people are laughing. Keep that image firmly in your mind for a few minutes. Then just relax and let your mind wander again. Every day 'tune in' to that person – he or she is *you*!

2. Let your imagination run riot when you read magazines and go to the cinema. Picture yourself in the glamorous clothes worn by the fashion models or the actors. Imagine yourself in exciting situations. Things only happen if you allow yourself to believe that it is a possibility that they might.

3. Take a fresh look at yourself. Julie had a 'make-over' – you can too. Have a new hair-cut, get some advice on make-up, ask your closest friends how they see you. If you are overweight, the chances are that you dress conservatively. It isn't necessary to do so. Don't wait until you are reed-slim, revamp your wardrobe now by buying one or two cheap bright items.

SUPPORT

The Fatfield slimmers were lucky because they had the support of friends, relatives, myself and my assistant, Toni, during their slimming and fitness campaign. The village, and surrounding area, is full of warm, charming people who love to get together. Families like John, Anne and Debbie Herkes encouraged each other to stay the course. Relatives like Julie Mulvaney and her sister-in-law Vera Churnside, provided mutual support. Whole groups of slimmers turned out to events like aquarobics sessions at the local pool and aerobics and weight-training classes.

At every weigh-in, there was a family party atmosphere. Slimmers were encouraged to bring friends and children along too. While advice was given privately if needed, slimmers could also involve their husbands and wives in the proceedings if they wished. There were strictly no penalties for not losing weight, just bags of encouragement all the way. One of the most important pieces of advice we gave our slimmers was to aim *low*: to think about the first half-stone, then the next . . . and so on.

Although it is obviously a tremendous advantage, and highly unusual, to get this degree of help while you slim, there are other ways to get support. Here are some ideas:

1. *Slim with your partner.* If you help your husband, wife or lover to lose a stone or two, and do the same yourself, it will strengthen your relationship. Be strong for them when their willpower wavers, praise their success, and take regular exercise together. Aim to be a glamorous, slim couple on that next holiday abroad, or for a special night out. It is important to be positive, so never nag!

2. *Slim with some friends.* Form a group – at work, with neighbours, or at the pub. Get together, follow the

Fatfield Diet, and raise some cash for a local good cause. It will be great fun and make the going easier. It is important to make sure that all group members check with their doctors before joining in.

3. *Be your own Slimming Counsellor.* If you prefer to go it alone, you can still get loads of encouragement – from yourself. Be your own best friend throughout your slim-in. Weigh yourself once a week, on the same scales, and keep a record of your progress. Keep that awful old photograph of yourself in an album, and get a friend to take regular Polaroid snaps of the new, emerging you. Gloat unashamedly at the improvement. Reward yourself with a new paperback, a trip to the cinema, or a couple of hours spent listening to music.

4. *Join our Fatfield Slim Pals.* While we were helping the Fatfield slimmers, we established a nationwide network of slimmers who keep in touch with each other by letter and telephone. We have matched up people with similar problems, so they can be mutually supportive. In some cases, our Slim Pals have met, exchanged views on slimming, and become firm friends. If you think you would benefit from chatting or writing to someone who is trying to lose weight, write to me at the address below, enclosing a stamped, addressed envelope and brief details about yourself, and your weight problems. We will send you full details about the Bazaar Fatfield Slim Pals scheme.

Write to: Bazaar Fatfield Slim Pals, c/o Sally Ann Voak, PO Box 618, Coulsdon, Surrey, CR5 1RU

CHAPTER EIGHT

THE FATFIELD
WORKOUT

We all know that exercise is good for us but most of us are too lazy to get out of our armchairs and go jogging, swimming or even for a brisk walk. Despite the boom in exercise tapes and videos, fitness classes, and sports clubs, the vast majority of people would still rather read about people exercising, or watch them doing it on television, than work out themselves. There are many overweight, unfit people who boast a whole shelf full of exercise videos, but have never tried to follow any of them.

Back in January 1991, when we started our fitness campaign, the residents of the little village of Fatfield were, like most of us, keen on thinking about exercise, but not so keen on doing any. But as the weight dropped off, they became much more fitness-conscious. Luckily for them, they had a highly qualified local fitness teacher, Susan Collins, to guide them. Susan runs classes in just about every form of exercise, from aquarobics to weight-training. Her base is the local community centre, and her classes are reasonably priced and always great fun.

The experience of Fatfield has proved to me that the best way to exercise is to start gently with swimming, walking and sitting-down routines, and work up to more vigorous sessions as you improve. Indeed, if you are a very overweight person, it is essential to take things very easily at first. Even if you are only a stone or so above your ideal weight, it is madness to leap into a vigorous aerobics class or go for 4-mile jogs every night if you are not used to it. You will end up with pulled muscles, possible back troubles, injuries to your joints or even a heart attack.

Our slimmers began with gentle aquarobics (exercises in water), swimming, simple stretching exercises, isometrics (exercises where the muscle is contracted through pushing, pulling, squeezing or pressing against an immovable object), and 'couch potato' exercises performed while watching television. Some found that they obtained a good level of fitness for their lifestyle with just one or two of the above. Some progressed to aerobics sessions, and even weight-training. I am proud to say that a few became so fit that they managed to survive a gruelling army assault course.

I have to admit that the Fatfield slimmers put me to shame. I gave up trying to fit exercise classes into my life some time ago, but I have always done isometric and 'couch potato' exercises while I work and watch television, and I try to break off work for a few stretching exercises a couple of times a day. I walk for miles at weekends, and occasionally treat myself to a course of toning table exercises, which are very effective indeed and involve the minimum of time and effort. In just one hour, you relax on six or eight different mechanical tables, which make your muscles work fairly hard while you simply breathe and move correctly. You feel refreshed afterwards but you do not look dishevelled and the inches do gradually come off, especially if you combine the course with one of the Fatfield diet plans.

The amount of fun obtained from exercise is of paramount importance. It is no earthly good doing any fitness routine unless you enjoy it. You may shape up your body but you are also likely to develop a harassed expression, frown lines, a droopy chest and a terrible passion for comfort foods.

Here are five great routines for lazy people like me and the Fatfield slimmers. They are all very easy, take up little time, and (most important) are safe for people on a slimming diet. At the end of the day, there really is no point in being super-fit unless you are an Olympic athlete. It is much better to achieve a level of fitness that helps you cope with the demands of your own lifestyle and guards against heart disease. That means you need a brisk workout three times a week which lasts 20 minutes, or longer, plus individual exercises to tone up the bits of you that wobble about.

AQUAROBICS AND BATH EXERCISES

Water is the ideal medium for exercise, especially if you are tense or tired, recovering from illness or injury, or are overweight.

It helps you exercise in two important ways: first, the pressure of water against your body (its resistance) helps you to build up strength gradually – you have to exert your muscles to get through the water. Second, its buoyancy supports the weight of your body, relieving the pressure of gravity on your spine and allowing the muscles of your legs and back (which usually have to work very hard to keep you standing up) to relax.

If you are a 'plumpie' who is shy about revealing your body in a swimsuit, you can either go to the pool in the early morning or throw caution to the wind and join a class.

Our intrepid Fatfield slimmers found that the hilarity of one of Susan's classes made them forget their wobbles and just have fun. If you can find a similar class in your area, do go along and join in – you could find that there are many people who are a lot fatter than you.

Try these in your local pool:

1. *Warm-up* Have a good splash about to get your circulation going. At waist-depth, jump repeatedly in all directions. Fling out your arms when you are at the top of the jump and keep your tummy muscles taught throughout.

2. *For spine, ankles, legs* With the water at waist level or deeper, face the side of the bath and hold it with both hands, about 3 feet (1 metre) apart. Now, let your legs float up behind you and kick without letting your feet break the surface of the water, keeping your knees straight, and taking very small 'steps'. Repeat 10 times, increasing to 25.

3. *For chest, back, shoulders, arms* Stand in shoulder-depth water and extend your arms together in front of you, then pull them back to the open-arm position. Try to get your shoulder blades to touch at the back and keep your fingers open for maximum 'drag'. Repeat 10 times, increasing to 25.

4. *For waist, side muscles, thighs, knees, arms* Stand with your feet wide apart in midriff-depth water. Now let your arms float on top of the water in front of you, and twist to the left and the right from your waist, using your arms as 'oars', and going as far as is comfortable with each swing. Repeat 10 times, increasing to 25.

5. *For bottom, hips and thighs* Stand waist-deep in the water, with legs comfortably apart, hands on your hips.

Jump to bring your feet together. Repeat 5 times, increasing to 20, when you get the hang of it.

6. *For legs, posture, balance* Still with water at waist-level, raise your hands straight out in front of you, palms down, and walk backwards through the water for a few steps. Walk forwards again. Repeat 5 times, trying to keep your balance and posture perfect.

Try these movements in the bath
You will get the same advantages as you do with aquarobics in the pool, with the added bonus of being able to do the exercises nude and in private. A bath pillow is essential, so you can relax while you work out.

1. *For tummy, thighs and lower back muscles* Lie back in the bath, arms by your sides, feet together, head resting comfortably on the bath pillow. Now, slowly raise your arms to the horizontal position, bending your knees and raising your feet off the bottom of the bath at the same time. Point your toes, hold the position for a count of 6, then lower feet and arms slowly. Repeat 5 times, increasing to 10.

2. *For tummy, legs, hips, shoulders, arms* Lie back in the bath, legs stretched out and toes wedged firmly under the taps, hands by your sides. Sit up slowly and stretch your arms to try and touch your toes, gently curl forward so your face comes down towards the water if you can. Hold for a count of 3, then relax back slowly. Repeat twice, increasing to 6 times.

3. *For tummy* Lie back again, feet resting on the bottom of the bath, knees bent, hands floating by your sides. Now pull in your tummy muscles, almost as though you were trying to touch your spine with your navel. Hold for a

count of 3 then relax. Repeat 5 times, resting between each exercise. Breathing is important here: breathe out deeply before you pull in your tummy muscles, breathe in again as you release them.

4. *For waist* Sit up in the bath, resting your feet on the bottom, legs slightly apart. Clasp your hands behind your head, making sure your back is straight, head held high. Twist your trunk slowly to the right, going as far as is comfortably possible. Hold for a count of 3, then return to starting position, and relax for a further count of 3. Repeat, twisting to the left this time. Repeat the whole movement 10 times.

WALKING

Walking just has to be the most underestimated form of exercise. It is free, easy, enjoyable and something we all do (although some of us try to avoid it as much as possible). Yet, it has never really caught on as a serious form of exercise.

Regular walking really can do a great deal to help you slim down and shape up your body. For a start, it uses up energy in a positive way. While you are walking, you are burning off calories at the rate of about six a minute. That might not sound much but it soon adds up. What's more, walking 'revs' up your metabolism and helps you burn off calories more quickly. This effect carries on, even when you stop walking. Contrary to what most people imagine, walking suppresses hunger pangs so, unless you plan your daily excursion to take in the local baker's, sweetshop, and fish and chip shop, you will be less likely to eat the wrong foods. It also gives you the mental relaxation you need to combat problems like stress and depression, which can also make you eat the wrong things.

Most important, walking makes you physically healthier and improves your looks by reducing fat and adding lean tissue at the same time. Some years ago, an interesting American study compared three groups of women. The first group cut back their daily food intake by 500 calories. The women in the second group ate the same amount as usual, but took enough exercise to burn off 500 calories daily. The third group did half and half, cutting back on 250 calories daily, and taking enough exercise to burn off another 250. The exercisers all worked out by walking on a treadmill. At the end of 16 weeks, the women had all lost roughly the same amount of weight, between $10^1/_2$ and $12^1/_2$lb each. But, the women who had taken exercise reshaped their bodies – losing more body fat (about $12^1/_2$lb) and gaining lean tissue. So, if you want your diet to work brilliantly and you also want to look firmer and leaner afterwards, follow the Fatfield Diet and *walk* your way to fitness. Here are six ways to do it:

1. *Leave the car at home.* You really do not need to drive to the corner shop, or to visit a friend a couple of streets away. It is a pleasure, more environmentally aware, and often quicker, to walk. Aim for a brisk, half-hour walk every single day.

2. *Choose an interesting spot.* Select a fascinating stretch of town, or a pretty walk in the country to be your very own walking route. Time yourself as you walk it, aiming to increase your pace from the normal human walking pace of between 3 and 4 miles an hour.

3. *Wear comfortable shoes.* You will never enjoy walking if your feet are killing you. Wear well-fitting sports shoes or trainers with good arch and ankle support, or low-heeled shoes or boots that do not rub or pinch.

4. *Walk with a friend*. It doesn't matter whether your chum is a lover, dog, or child, you will both get a big kick out of walking together, away from the pressures of your family, work or television set.

5. *Step out indoors*. Crazy though it sounds, you probably do most of your walking inside your own home. The trouble is that normally you do not walk briskly enough for it to do very much good. Try hotting up the action, by dashing up and down stairs, walking on the spot while you watch a lunchtime television show, or even using the bottom step of the stairs for some 'stepping'. This is the hot 'new' exercise rave in America, and simply consists of stepping up and down on a portable platform. Your own front doorstep is just as good.

6. *Be a happy hiker*. The cheapest way to have fun at weekends is to take a bus into the country, and go for a ramble. It may sound old-fashioned but it does wonderful things for your shape and for your bank balance. What's more, you see something of the countryside, instead of just whizzing through it in a car. All you need are stout shoes, a hooded waterproof jacket and some low-calorie sandwiches from your Fatfield Diet plan.

ISOMETRICS

If you want to work your muscles hard without any huffing and puffing, try these exercises. They are isometrics, and the muscle is contracted through pushing, pulling, squeezing or pressing against an immovable object. The force of resistance acts as pressure and the muscle is made to work very hard, promoting strength, tone and endurance.

The beauty of these exercises is that you can do them at home, at work, or even while travelling.

1. *For inside thigh muscles* Sit comfortably with your back straight and shoulders relaxed. Now place a suitably sturdy object such as a briefcase or metal wastepaper basket, between your feet. Squeeze your feet together as hard as possible for a count of 10, then relax. Repeat 10 times.

2. *For upper arms* Sit with your back straight, feet together, shoulders relaxed, and place the palms of your hands on a table or desk in front of you. Now press down as hard as you can, as if you were trying to force the table down. Hold the position for a count of 6. Relax. Now put your hands just under the table, palms up, elbows tucked in. Push up as hard as you can, hold for a count of 6, then relax. Repeat each movement 5 times.

3. *For upper back and tummy muscles* Sit with your back straight, feet slightly apart, palms of your hands flat on your thighs. Keeping your arms perfectly straight, take a breath, then exhale as you press down, pulling in your tummy muscles at the same time. Hold for a count of 6, then relax. Inhale and repeat 5 times.

4. *For chest muscles* Sitting in your car (while parked!) or at your desk, grip the steering wheel at the nine o'clock and three o'clock positions or place the palms of your hands against the sides of your computer terminal or typewriter. Now push hard with elbows tucked in (women should see their bosom 'jump' slightly), hold for a count of 6, then relax. Repeat 5 times.

COUCH POTATO EXERCISES

If you watch television for three or four hours every evening, it makes sense to combine your viewing with some easy exercises. Do them during the boring bits, or the commercials. It is a good idea to sit on a firm chair for one of the exercises, although you can do most of them sitting on the sofa.

1. *For shoulders* Sit with your back straight, feet slightly apart, hands clasped loosely behind you with elbows slightly bent. Now draw your shoulder blades together, and push your upper arms together, without trying to straighten your arms. Repeat 6 times.

2. *For bottom* Sit with your back straight, feet slightly apart and forward with knees slightly bent. Place the palms of your hands on your upper chest and relax your shoulders. Now contract your thigh muscles hard, and rotate them outwards. You should feel your buttock muscles contracting. Relax and repeat 6 times.

3. *For waistline* Sit with your back straight, the palms of your hands on your upper chest. Now lift your breastbone and rib-cage and twist your torso and head around to the left as far as you can with your pelvis still facing forwards. Now twist just a little more in short, sharp movements. Return to face the front and repeat to the right. Repeat 6 times each way.

4. *For tummy and pelvis* Sit near the front of a straight-backed chair for this one. Your feet should be flat on the floor, knees slightly apart, and you should grasp the seat of the chair near the back. Now, keeping your back straight, inhale, then exhale as you tilt your pelvis up so the pubic bone rises but your bottom stays put, in a rolling movement. The curve of your lower spine will straighten and your tummy will be pulled in. Relax and repeat 10 times.

5. *For bust* Sit with your knees slightly apart, shoulders relaxed, back straight. Now clench your fists and bring your arms upwards strongly, elbows bent, so they cross

over in front of you. Repeat this 'scissors' movement 20 times.

6. *For legs* Sorry, for this one you have got to get off the sofa and lie down on the carpet, but you can still carry on watching your favourite programme. Lie on your right side with your body and legs in a straight line. Prop your head on your right hand with your left hand on the floor in front of you for balance. With your foot flexed (the toe pointing forwards), raise your leg as high as you can comfortably do so. Pause briefly, then lower it to about 10 inches off the floor. Repeat 5 times, swap sides and repeat. (While you are facing away from the television set, get your family to fill you in on the action!)

STRETCHING EXERCISES

These are excellent exercises to do in the middle of the day, or when you get home from work. They help you unwind your body, particularly if it has been confined behind a bench, desk or driving wheel all day long. It is essential to do them in a warm room, wearing loose clothing, and to start off very gently. These six exercises are based on yoga *asanas* which are wonderful for helping to banish stress, improve concentration, and relieve depression and anxiety. I do recommend slimmers to try yoga, particularly those who eat the wrong things when they are under pressure.

1. *Relaxation* Lie on your back on the floor with your legs slightly apart, hands a little way from your body, palms uppermost. Now, let your feet flop open and close your eyes, breathing quietly and evenly. Allow yourself two or three minutes of complete relaxation, then open your eyes, and get up slowly.

2. *For tummy and thighs* Kneel with your back straight, head erect and arms relaxed beside you. Take a deep breath, and hold it as you lean back, making sure your body and thighs stay in a straight line. Go just a little way at first. Hold for a count of 2 then straighten up smoothly, breathing in as you do so. Repeat 4 times, then relax, sitting back on your heels.

3. *For spine, shoulder and neck muscles* Kneel on the floor and place your hands on the floor in front of you with hands shoulders' width apart. Breathing slowly and normally throughout the movement, hollow your back and look up at the ceiling. Count to 5, then reverse the position by arching your back and gently pushing your pelvis forward. Try to make your chin touch your chest. Count to 5 and repeat the entire movement twice. Rest, sitting back on your heels for a few moments, then repeat twice more.

4. *For spine, tummy and chest* Lie on your tummy on the floor. Bend your elbows and place the palms of your hands in front of you, fingertips touching, so you can rest your left cheek on the backs of your hands. Now take a breath and exhale as you press your hands down, straighten your arms and raising your upper body off the ground. Look up at the ceiling, count to 5, and relax down to the first position, breathing in as you do so. Repeat 3 times.

5. *For legs and ankles* Stand straight, head erect, legs and feet together. Now raise your arms in front of you to shoulder level, palms of your hands facing the floor. Keeping your back perfectly straight, take a breath, then exhale as you bend your knees and come up onto the balls of your feet. Go down as far as possible without wobbling. Now breathe in as you straighten up. Repeat 4 times.

6. *For back, legs, arms, tummy muscles* Stand, feet together, arms above your head, fingers clasped loosely.

Look up at your hands. Bend your knees and bring your hands down slowly to the horizontal position, with your knees bent. Let your hands fall sideways and down, and relax your head forward, bending your knees still further. Pause, then reverse the movement. Repeat 5 times. Breathe in as you raise your body, out as you lower it.

CHAPTER NINE

HOW TO KEEP WEIGHT OFF – THE FATFIELD WAY

One very important effect of the Fatfield Diet is that, once you stop slimming, weight does *not* creep back on easily. You really have to work at it!

Joking aside, it is quite difficult to eat much more than you are already eating on the diet. After you have tasted so much good, healthy, enjoyable food, it takes time to slip back into old habits. Fatty foods seem greasy and disgusting, over-cooked vegetables look unappetising, sugar in your tea tastes just awful. The diet re-trains your eating habits so well that you do not want to rush for a cream bun 'fix' as soon as you reach your goal weight.

It is well known that many slimming plans encourage you to put weight back on when you stop dieting. After weeks, or months of deprivation, your body is delighted when extra food arrives on the scene and promptly stores it – as fat. On the Fatfield Diet, calories are never cut down too much, and bulk is maintained all the way through. The result? Satisfaction not deprivation.

It is still too early to say whether all our Fatfield slimming guinea-pigs will keep off the weight they have lost on the diet. Several did reach their 'goal' during the slim-in and have kept off the weight very successfully indeed since then. One reason for this is that they all learned to enjoy exercising while they dieted and have kept up regular work-outs ever since. This helps keep their metabolism in 'top gear', so the fuel-burning processes have not become sluggish.

They also enjoyed the feeling of well-being produced by eating healthy foods instead of fat or sugar-loaded 'junk' food.

'I feel like a different person,' says Pam Orwin, 27, who lost 3 stone 4lb. Pam has a very busy life indeed. She has two young children, a part-time job as a barmaid and is also studying at college. 'Before I changed my eating habits, I was often tired and fed-up. Now, I look forward to each day. My college work is a terrific challenge, and I even find time to go to aerobics classes.'

Lynn Ayre, who was the first slimmer to shed 2 stone, and now weighs 11 stone 10lb, says, 'The big moment for me came when I bought a clingy, black Lycra dress in a size 14. It was the first time I had worn size 14 since my wedding day ten years ago. As soon as I put it on, and looked in the mirror, I vowed that I would *never* get fat again – and I won't!'

When you feel as good as that about yourself, it is crazy to go off the straight and narrow. But, guess what, I am now going to give you permission to do just that. Eating the wrong things, occasionally, is not a sin. What is important is how you deal with it. It is also important to find out just how many calories you can consume without putting on weight. The Fatfield Maintenance Plan on page 140 has been specially devised to help you work out your own best calorie intake level.

It gives a good basic diet, allowing about 1500 calories for women, 1800 for men. Follow it for two weeks after you finish your Fatfield Slimming Diet plan, and weigh in at the end of the two weeks. If you are still losing, add one of the 100 calorie Extras (which include sweet treats, more bread, and even a little more alcohol) to the plan and follow it for one more week.

If the pounds are still dropping off, add another 100 calorie Extra, follow the diet for a further week – and so on.

When you have established the perfect calorie level to maintain your weight, try to stick within that range. If you consume more calories one day, try to make up for it the next day by eating simple, healthy meals from our recipe section or the Basic Fatfield Plan with lots of green vegetables.

Here are your *Top Ten Rules* for staying in shape:

1. *Don't* panic if the scales show you have put on a few pounds. This could be caused by fluid retention, or a little over-indulgence. Calmly, go back on the basic Maintenance Diet, until the extra weight drops off again. At the same time, increase the amount of exercise you take. Just walking for an extra half-hour a day should do the trick.

2. *Don't* feel guilty if you eat chocolate, sweets or cakes. If you buy them furtively and wolf them down in secret, you will get a severe attack of guilt, which will make you crave *more* and could even lead to bingeing. Instead, enjoy your treat, eating it slowly and savouring every single mouthful. Make a mental note of the calories the treat contains and make sure you trim off the same amount from your next day's calorie total.

3. *Do* throw out your old clothes or alter them to fit your new shape. If you keep a wardrobe which consists of 'fat' and 'thin' outfits, you are programming yourself, mentally,

to pile on pounds again. Remember, you are a slim person now, so you do not need large-size clothes any more.

4. *Don't* eat too little. You might be tempted to slip back into bad old habits like eating very little during the first half of the day, then snacking all evening. It is very dangerous indeed to do this. Concentrate on maintaining a healthy food intake at all times.

5. *Do* show off your new body. It is very hard to become adjusted to a new, slim shape. Increase your self-confidence by going out and about much more than you did when you were fatter. Go for those goals we talked about on page 114. Wear shorts, join a hang-gliding club, sunbathe in a tiny swimsuit. Get your partner or a friend to take some good photographs of you, so you can keep your own *Before and After* record of your slimming achievement. Vanity is healthy, so keep right on admiring yourself and even buy a few new mirrors so you can really enjoy the view.

6. *Do* keep busy. One of the best bits of advice for anyone who wants to stay slim is to be too busy – with work, hobbies, and projects – to crave high-fat and high-carbohydrate snacks. If you are working full-time, cram some fitness or vocational evening classes into the day. If you are working part-time or not at all, join a club, help with your favourite charity, or plunge yourself into a task like redecorating the house or landscaping the garden.

7. *Do* be extra loving to your partner. Some slimmers find that their 'other half', intentionally or unintentionally, tries to sabotage all their efforts to stay slim by encouraging them to eat and drink the wrong things. Don't forget that it can be very upsetting to watch a familiar, well-rounded loved one change into a slim, dynamic person.

Naturally, your partner is bound to feel threatened by the new you. Be strong; show lots of love and concern, but refuse to allow the saboteur to pile up cheesecake on your plate, or pour you another large Scotch. Don't forget, *you* (and *only* you) are in charge of your own body!

8. *Do* become a Fatfield Supercook. Collect recipes and meal ideas which will enlarge your repertoire of huge, satisfying, low-fat high-fibre meals. Try out ways of cooking exotic dishes using the Fatfield principles described on page 39. Italian, Chinese, Mexican and French dishes can all be prepared the Fatfield way, by subtly changing ingredients and cooking methods.

9. *Do* write and tell me how you are getting on. We want as much information as possible about the long-term success of the Fatfield Diet. So do drop me a line – with photographs if possible – to the address on page 121. Do enclose a stamped, addressed envelope.

10. *Do* tell your friends how you lost weight. The more you can spread the word about the Fatfield Diet, the better. Once you have built up a reputation as a successful slimmer, you will have all the more reason for staying slim. Even better, start your own group of Fatfield Slimmers with yourself as leader. For a leaflet on forming a group, do write to me – again at the address on page 121. The leaflet is free, but I would like you to send a stamped, addressed envelope. Thanks!

HEALTHY EATING IS A WAY OF LIFE

If you follow the Maintenance Plan on the next page, you'll have a blueprint for healthy eating – and for life. It contains all the goodies you need to help you stay slim, trim, and full of vitality.

You can adapt the plan to fit in with your life style so

long as you shop and cook wisely following the advice in this book. As the months go by, you'll reap the rewards of good nutrition with extra energy, fewer health problems, and lots more fun!

THE FATFIELD MAINTENANCE PLAN

EVERY DAY ³/₄ pint (425ml) skimmed milk for your tea and coffee, unlimited water, mineral water and diet soft drinks. Use an artificial sweetener such as Hermestas instead of sugar.

MEN Add 2 slices wholemeal bread or a medium wholemeal roll with a little low-fat spread, plus 1 glass dry wine or ¹/₂ pint beer or lager.

FREE VEGETABLES Choose them from the list on page 35.

CALORIES About 1500 calories for women, 1800 for men. You may add calories (as explained above) by choosing items from the 100 calorie Extras list below.

BREAKFAST (choose *one*, packed if necessary)

- ¹/₂ grapefruit, with sweetener, 1oz (25g) any unsweetened cereal with milk from allowance, 1 slice wholemeal toast topped with 2 tsp honey or marmalade
- 1 slice wholemeal toast with 1 size 3 poached egg, half 5oz (125g) can baked beans, 1 large banana
- 1 Shredded Wheat biscuit, milk from allowance, 1 carton Diet Ski yogurt, 1 slice wholemeal toast with a little low-fat spread, 1 apple or pear
- Sandwich of 2 slices wholemeal bread with filling of 1 cooked low-fat sausage, mustard or 1 tsp tomato ketchup, 1 apple or orange

- 1 medium wholemeal roll with filling of 1 rasher well-grilled back bacon, grilled tomatoes, 5 fl oz (125ml) unsweetened fruit juice, 1 satsuma
- 2oz (50g) unsweetened muesli, milk from allowance, 1 chopped apple, 1 small carton natural yogurt
- 1 pot Golden Wonder Pot Noodles, any flavour, a few grapes
- 1 slice wholemeal toast topped with small (7.6oz/215g) can Heinz Spaghetti in Tomato Sauce, grilled tomatoes, 1 small banana

LUNCHES (choose *one*)

Sandwich made with 2 slices wholemeal bread or a medium sized wholemeal or granary roll with one of the following fillings and accompaniments:

- 1oz (25g) any hard cheese, 1 Diet Ski yogurt, 1 banana
- 2oz (50g) lean ham or chicken (no skin), 1 mug Batchelors Slim a Soup, 1 apple, orange or pear
- 1 well-grilled low-fat sausage, 1 tsp sweet pickle, 1 carton Shape Fromage Frais
- 1 pot Shippam's Paste, any flavour, 1 small carton cottage cheese with pineapple
- 1 pot Shape Low-Fat Soft Cheese, any flavour, 1 Harvest Crunch Bar

Do not forget to pile on the 'free' salad and vegetables, either in your sandwich or roll, or as a separate dish, packed in a sealed container to keep it crisp.

OR
One meal chosen from this list:

- 1 slice of melon, 6oz (150g) any grilled or steamed white fish, 5oz (125g) jacket potato, 1 apple or pear

- 1 well-grilled beefburger, 3oz (75g) oven chips, 1 orange
- 2 slices wholemeal toast topped with one of the following: 1 small can (5oz/125g) baked beans, 1 small can Heinz Wholewheat Spaghetti in Tomato Sauce, 1 poached egg. Followed by 1 apple or orange, and 1 digestive biscuit
- 6oz (150g) jacket potato, topped with 4oz (100g) chopped cooked chicken with 1 tbsp low-calorie salad cream, 1 apple
- 1 large slice of melon, 10oz (250g) chicken leg (no skin) grilled or roast, 1 small wholemeal roll with a little low-fat spread

Please do not forget your 'free' vegetables and salad.

SUPPERS (choose *one*)

Any of the suppers in the Basic Plan on page 46, plus 1 apple, orange or small banana.

OR
One of these:

- Any Findus Lean Cuisine ready meal with 5oz (125g) jacket potato
- 1 can (6oz/150g) John West Pilchards in Tomato Sauce with 3oz (75g) mashed potato, made up with milk from allowance, 2 crispbreads with a little low-fat spread
- 1 portion Kentucky Fried Chicken, 1 portion coleslaw, 1 apple or orange
- 1 McDonald's Cheeseburger, or 6 Chicken McNuggets, regular orange juice
- $1/_2$ thin crust medium pizza from a pizza restaurant or takeaway, 1 apple or orange to follow

- Restaurant meal of melon or clear soup, simply-cooked fish or lean meat (no sauces), medium jacket potato

TREATS (choose *one* each day)

- 1 extra apple or orange
- 1 Jaffa Cake
- 1 After Eight Mint
- 1 small wholemeal roll with salad filling
- 1 mug Batchelors Slim a Soup with 1 crispbread
- 1 Ferrero Rocher chocolate
- 1 Rowntree Rolo
- 1 Diet Ski yogurt, any flavour

ALCOHOL
You may have ¹/₂ pint beer, lager or stout, or 1 glass dry wine or sherry, or 2 pub-measure 'short' drinks with low-calorie mixers.

100 CALORIE EXTRAS

- 1 slice wholemeal bread with a little low-fat spread
- 2oz (50g) (no skin) chicken, or ham (lean only), or lean beef, lamb or pork. In practice, that is an extra *thin* slice at dinner or suppertime.
- 4oz (100g) poached or grilled white fish with no fat added, or 3oz (75g) shellfish, again cooked without fat or sauces
- 2oz (50g) chunk roast potato, or 3oz (75g) potato, mashed with milk from your allowance
- 4oz (100g) peas, beans or sweetcorn
- ¹/₂ pint beer, lager or stout, or 1 glass dry wine, or 2 pub-measure 'short' drinks with low-calorie mixers.

In Part Two, you'll find a huge
selection of recipes which have been
specially created to help you enjoy your diet.
They are all low in calories, yet they are
tasty, satisfying and the portion sizes
are very generous indeed.

Each recipe has been calorie counted,
so it's easy to fit them into your Fatfield
plan. Remember, if you are following one of
the lower-calorie diets (e.g. the Quick
Weight Loss or the Anti-Bloating Plan), then
choose the lower-calorie recipes. Slimmers
who are on the higher-calorie plans (e.g. the
Heavy-Duty or the Boozers' Plan) can afford
to pick the more calorific dishes.

Vary your daily menus as much
as possible to ensure good nutrition and
plenty of surprises to tickle your taste buds
– that's the secret of successful slimming!

PART TWO

THE RECIPES

USING THE RECIPES

Every recipe in this book is simple to prepare.

- First, read through the ingredients and step-by-step preparation and cooking methods. Next, check your storecupboard, fridge or freezer for ingredients already available.

- When shopping, take the book with you, so you have a handy list in your basket.

- Work through each step carefully, and you are guaranteed success.

Recipe Notes

- Measurements are given both in imperial and metric amounts, but follow one set of measurements only.

- All spoon measures are level. If you use heaped spoonfuls remember the calorie counts will alter! One tablespoon (tbsp) = 15ml, one dessertspoon (dsp) = 10ml and one teaspoon (tsp) = 5ml.

- Ovens should always be preheated to the specified temperature.

- Eggs are size 3 or medium unless the recipe says otherwise.

- Use freshly ground black pepper when the recipe calls for pepper.

CHAPTER TEN

BASIC RECIPES

In this chapter is a selection of basic Fatfield recipes to get you started. You will find here lots of the recipes which are referred to in the Diet Plans. There are recipes for both family suppers and dinner parties, as well as new exciting ways to cook vegetables, essential sauces, and mouthwatering desserts.

The recipes are divided into the following sections:

STARTERS
CITRUS SALAD IN YOGURT DRESSING

Serves: 4
Calories per serving: 107

This is light and delicious. A perfect summer starter, and a scrumptious breakfast too.

2 medium oranges
2 medium grapefruit
20 green grapes
2 tbsp finely chopped fresh mint leaves
1 carton Shape Natural Yogurt
mint sprigs and 1 kiwi fruit to garnish

1.   Grate the zest from 1 orange. Place in a bowl.
2.   Remove all peel and pith from the oranges and grapefruit and discard. Halve grapes and remove pips. Then, over the bowl, carefully cut between membranes to remove citrus fruit segments.
3.   Add chopped mint and yogurt to the grated zest, oranges, grapefruit and grapes in the bowl. Leave in the refrigerator to marinate. Serve garnished with mint leaves and sliced kiwi fruit.

GREEK VEGETABLE SOUP

Serves: 4
Calories per serving: 76

Tasty and filling, this makes a good starter for a dinner party and is excellent for a family supper too. The tangy taste makes you think of balmy Mediterranean nights eating out under the stars.

15fl oz (425ml) canned consommé
4oz (100g) frozen mixed vegetables
10fl oz (275ml) natural unsweetened yogurt
1 egg yolk
1 tbsp chopped fresh mint
grated zest of $^1/_2$ lemon

1.   Heat the soup with the vegetables, cover and simmer for 10 minutes.
2.   Beat the yogurt with the egg yolk and gradually stir in some of the hot soup. Return to the pan and mix well until hot, but not boiling.
3.   Serve sprinkled with herbs and lemon zest.

TONI'S MACKEREL AND LEMON PATÉ

Serves: 4
Calories per serving: 155

This tasty and normally high-calorie paté is delicious with crispbreads or Nimble toast. Serve for breakfast, lunch or as a starter.

6oz (175g) fillet smoked mackerel
5.3oz (150g) carton Shape low-fat soft cream cheese
1 tbsp lemon juice
1 tsp creamed horseradish sauce
freshly ground black pepper

1.   Remove the skin and any bones from the mackerel. Mash all the ingredients together with a fork for a rough paté, or mix together with an electric mixer for a smooth paté.
2.   Divide into 4 individual bowls or ramekin dishes.

BEFORE

Russell and Vera Churnside look years younger now than they did when they started the Fatfield Diet. They feel full of energy, too. Vera, 30, who lost 6lb, goes to seven fitness classes each week, and has recently taken up horse-riding. Russell, 32, lost 17lb. He recently tried hang-gliding for the first time. 'We both feel tons fitter,' says Vera, 'and our three young daughters are delighted with their new mum and dad.

'One of the best things about the diet is that you eat so much delicious food,' she says. 'It fits in easily with our family life, and it is economical too.'

AFTER

BEFORE

AFTER

Erika Lowdon (*in the foreground, above*), who lost 24lb, has her husband, Austin, to thank for providing the fresh vegetables she enjoys on the diet. 'Austin grows broccoli, cabbage, leeks, onions – you name it – on his allotment, which adjoins our garden. I can cook up the most wonderful vegetable dishes, knowing that I can eat as much as I like.'

Erika, 63, underwent serious surgery during the Fatfield Diet experiment, and is certain that healthy eating helped her recovery. 'I feel strongly that everyone should try to improve their eating habits after a stay in hospital,' she says.

BEFORE

Lynn Ayre lost 45lb, and is so thrilled that she has become a Fatfield Slim Pal counsellor – helping another mum with a big weight problem to shed her excess pounds, by encouraging her with regular telephone calls.

The 28-year-old mother-of-two is still following the diet, and hopes to lose at least another 2 stone. She says: 'A few months ago, I was hardly the ideal person to help someone lose weight. Now, I have so much more confidence in myself. My biggest thrill was to put on a pair of jeans with a size 32-inch-waist for the first time. Now, they are loose!'

AFTER

Janine, 32, is a busy mother *and* a talented dancer. She was just a little overweight when she started the Fatfield Diet, weighing in at 9st 8lb (she's 5ft tall). 'My problem was that I felt so tired and run down,' she says. 'I was eating very little apart from chocolate biscuits! My face was puffy, and I had wobbly hips and thighs.'

At first, she actually *gained* weight, but now she is a trim 9st 1lb, which is fine for a dancer, and looks absolutely great. 'I am very pleased that I no longer feel so exhausted all the time,' she says. 'I think that my dancing has improved, too.'

BEFORE

AFTER

BEFORE

AFTER

John and Ann Herkes (*pictured above with their daughter, Debbie*) lost a total of 30lb between them, and are delighted with their new image. John, 56, gave up smoking during our Fatfield slim-in, but was still able to stick to the diet:

'The fact that you are allowed to nibble the "free" vegetables all day really helps former smokers like me,' he says. 'It stopped me from reaching for comfort foods as a cigarette substitute.'

His wife, Ann, is now changing her fashion image to suit her new shape. 'I can now wear much younger-looking clothes,' she says.

BEFORE

Brenda Taylor, 37, shed 31lb, and is still losing. She works shifts, but found that the diet can be easily adapted to fit in with the most awkward working hours. 'My daughter and husband love the recipes,' she says. 'I couldn't follow a diet where the meals weren't suitable for the whole family.'

Brenda is now able to wear much trendier clothes and has taken up horse-riding with her Fatfield neighbour, Vera Churnside. 'Six months ago I would never have dreamed of such an adventurous hobby,' she says. 'I am having so much fun now that I have lost weight.'

AFTER

BEFORE

AFTER

Susan Smith had so many food allergies that she feared that she wouldn't be able to follow a slimming diet. But we were able to tailor the basic Fatfield plan to suit her – and she has now lost 19lb.

Slimmers who have similar problems should show the Diet to their doctor or hospital dietician before starting.

Susan, 36, says: 'The diet has definitely helped reduce my asthma attacks. Anyone who has ever taken steroid drugs will know how depressing the extra weight-gain can make you feel. This plan really has worked wonders for me.'

Photograph: Mark Pepper

The Fatfield slimmers were so thrilled with their weight-loss (a total of 60st 2lb), that they decided to rename the village!

'After' photographs by *The Sun* newspaper, Steve Lewis

FRENCH ONION SOUP

Serves: 4
Calories per serving: 150

This very low-calorie soup is ideal to use as a 'filler'. Make up a batch and have some before your supper or before you go out for the evening—it helps to curb your appetite. Don't be put off by the bread and cheese—it is low in calories. Really!

1lb (450g) large onions, finely chopped
1 beef stock cube
1 pint (575ml) water
1 tbsp brandy (for special occasions)
4oz (100g) piece of French bread
1oz (25g) Edam cheese, grated

1.   Add the finely chopped onions to the water and stock cube, bring to the boil, and cook until soft. Simmer for 20 minutes.
2.   Remove some of the onions and put the soup and the rest of the onions through a blender. Return to the saucepan and heat through with the brandy if using it.
3.   Divide into 4 bowls. Add the reserved onions to the soup.
4.   In each bowl, add a 1oz piece (25g) of French bread and sprinkle with a quarter of the cheese. Place under the grill until the cheese has melted and the bread is soaked with soup.

SUPPERS
SPAGHETTI CARBONARA

Serves: 4
Calories per serving: 450

This traditional Italian favourite has had its calories trimmed so that it is suitable for slimmers with a taste for something sumptuous.

10oz (275g) (dry weight) spaghetti
6 rashers streaky bacon
2oz (50g) Shape Mature type cheddar
2 size 3 eggs
$^1/_4$ pint (150ml) Shape Single

1.   Cook the spaghetti in boiling salted water.
2.   Thoroughly grill the bacon and chop roughly.
3.   Grate the cheese and beat the eggs.
4.   Drain the spaghetti and return to the pan away from the heat. Add the bacon, Shape Single, egg and most of the cheese. Stir well to coat the spaghetti—the heat of the spaghetti will cook the eggs. Place in a hot serving dish and sprinkle with the remaining cheese.

STEAK AND KIDNEY CASSEROLE

Serves: 4
Calories per serving: 375 (includes rice)

A hearty family supper dish, or a Sunday 'special', this has the traditional taste without the fatty bits!

12oz (350g) stewing steak
6oz (175g) kidney
$1/_2$oz (15g) low-fat spread
1 large onion
8oz (225g) mushrooms
1 pint (575ml) beef stock
1 tsp tomato purée
dash Worcestershire sauce
salt and pepper
2oz (50g) (dry weight) rice per person

1.   Discard all visible fat from the cubed steak and kidney and place in a casserole dish. Add the finely chopped onion and the mushrooms, beef stock, tomato purée, a dash of Worcestershire sauce and salt and pepper.
2.   Cook in the oven at 170°C, 325°F or gas mark 3 until the beef is tender (about 2 hours).
3.   Cook the rice and serve with the casserole.

PORK PAPRIKA

Serves: 4
Calories per serving: 260

The paprika, onion and yogurt add an exotic touch to these delicious pork chops. This is a good dinner party choice as it is very easy to prepare, yet looks spectacular.

4 lean boneless pork chops (about 6oz/175g each)
salt and pepper
1 onion, chopped
$^1/_2$ tbsp oil
1 tbsp paprika (or to taste)
$2^1/_2$oz (65g) canned tomato purée
5 fl oz (125ml) stock made from chicken stock cube
6oz (175g) small button mushrooms
10oz (275g) natural yogurt

1. Heat oven to 180°C, 350°F, gas mark 4.
2. Season pork chops and put under grill to seal on both sides. Remove from heat, cut off fat. Keep to one side.
3. In a flameproof casserole, gently cook onion in oil until soft. Blend in paprika and cook for a further minute. Add tomato purée. Remove from heat and blend in stock.
4. Return to heat and bring to the boil, stirring well. Taste and adjust seasoning. Add the pork chops. Cover and cook for 30 minutes or until meat is tender.
5. Five minutes before end of cooking time, add the mushrooms. Just before serving, spoon over the natural yogurt.

FISH CASSEROLE

Serves: 4
Calories per serving: 240

This reasonably priced casserole is a favourite for parties.

$1^1/_2$lb (675g) cod or coley fillet
1 clove garlic, chopped
1 large onion, finely sliced
1 tbsp olive oil
$^1/_2$oz (15g) low-fat spread
4 courgettes, washed and sliced
4oz (100g) mushrooms, peeled and sliced
4 tomatoes, skinned and chopped
2 tbsp tomato purée
7fl oz (200ml) water
dried basil
2oz (50g) black olives
4oz (100g) prawns or shrimps, peeled
salt and freshly ground black pepper
1 tbsp chopped parsley and 4–8 slices lemon for garnish

1.   Gently fry garlic and onion in olive oil and low-fat spread until translucent.
2.   Add courgettes, mushrooms, tomatoes, tomato purée, water, and basil. Season to taste. Cover and simmer for about 15 minutes.
3.   Add olives and prawns. Place fish in a heavy saucepan or casserole and pour sauce over it. Cover and simmer for 15–20 minutes until the fish is cooked.
4.   Garnish with freshly chopped parsley and slices of lemon and serve with 3oz (75g) peas and 4oz (100g) mashed potato.

FATFIELD BUBBLE AND SQUEAK

Serves: 4
Calories per serving: 300

This is one of the Fatfield village favourites and a good, low-calorie way of using up leftover vegetables. Great as a Monday night supper dish, served with a huge mixed salad.

8oz (225g) cooked greens
2lb (900g) cooked mashed potato
2 carrots, peeled and grated
1 large onion
pinch nutmeg
1 tsp sunflower oil
2 tbsp grated wholemeal breadcrumbs
1oz (25g) grated strong Cheddar cheese

1.   Chop the cooked greens and mix with the cooked mashed potato.
2.   Place the grated carrots, sliced onion, pinch of nutmeg, and a splash of water into a saucepan. Cover and cook over gentle heat for 4 minutes.
3.   Stir into the mashed potato mixture, and season.
4.   Heat 1 tsp sunflower oil in a non-stick frying pan over a medium heat, add the vegetable mixture and level the top. Cook over a medium heat until the underside is crisp and golden. When cooked place under a hot grill until the top is brown.
5.   Sprinkle the wholemeal breadcrumbs, and the grated cheese over the top and grill again until it is golden brown.

FATFIELD SHEPHERD'S PIE

Serves: 4
Calories per serving: 300

This pie is highly recommended by Rose Irwin, one of our successful Fatfield slimmers, who dishes this up for her family and herself. No-one ever complains about eating Mum's diet food!

8oz (225g) lean minced beef
2 large onions
$^1/_2$oz (15g) low-fat spread
2 tsps oil
1 large can (15oz/425g) baked beans
$^1/_4$ pint (150ml) beef stock
1lb (450g) potato, cooked and mashed

1.   Brown the minced beef in its own fat and drain on kitchen paper. Transfer to a pie plate
2.   Fry the chopped onions in the low-fat spread and oil. Transfer to the mince and mix in the can of baked beans, adding enough stock to make a moist consistency.
3.   Spread the mashed potato over the top, fluff up with a fork, bake in the oven for 40 minutes until golden. Serve with 'free' vegetables.

LIVER AND ONION GRAVY

Serves: 1
Calories per serving: 300

Liver is never dry and boring served with this delicious onion sauce. If you like the liver pink inside, cut down the cooking time by a minute or so.

1 small onion, finely chopped
$1/_4$ pint (150ml) beef stock
4oz (100g) lamb's liver
1 heaped tbsp skimmed milk powder
1 tsp cornflour

1.   In a large frying pan, fry the finely chopped onion until translucent. Add 2tbsp water and the beef stock cube and cook for 4 minutes.
2.   Cut the lamb's liver into $1/_4$-inch slices. Place on top of onions. Cover and cook for 10 minutes or until liver is tender. Remove meat from pan and keep warm.
3.   Add the skimmed milk powder to the cornflour and mix with 5 tbsp water. Stir into onion mixture and bring to the boil. Pour onion sauce over the liver. Serve with plenty of 'free' vegetables.

PIQUANT MINCE WITH DISHY DUMPLINGS

Serves: 4
Calories per serving: 320

Whoever heard of eating dumplings on a slimming diet? Well, this is no ordinary diet and these are no ordinary dumplings. They are boiling over with taste-appeal!

12oz (350g) lean mince
1 small onion, chopped
1 stick celery, thinly sliced
1 small carrot, diced
1 beef stock cube
2 tbsp tomato purée
dash Worcestershire sauce
1 bay leaf
Dumplings
3oz (75g) self-raising flour
pinch salt
$1^{1}/_{2}$oz (40g) vegetable suet

1.   Brown the mince in a non-stick pan and then drain off the fat. Place meat in a casserole dish.
2.   Add the thinly sliced celery, chopped onion and diced carrot to the casserole dish and mix with the minced beef.
3.   Dissolve the stock cube and tomato purée in 7fl oz (200ml) boiling water, and add to the casserole. Add the Worcestershire sauce and bay leaf. Cover and cook at 190°C, 375°F, gas mark 5 for 45 minutes.
4.   Sieve the self-raising flour with the salt and add the vegetable suet. Mix with enough water to make a firm dough. Shape into 4 dumplings and place on top of the meat. Cook for 25 minutes. Serve with 'free' vegetables.

BEEF WITH BEAN CASSEROLE

Serves: 4
Calories per serving: 250

Kidney beans help 'bulk out' this casserole, so it is less expensive than it looks. You can prepare this in advance and it freezes well, too.

12oz (350g) lean, cubed braising or stewing steak
1 tbsp sunflower oil
1 onion, sliced
1 green pepper, de-seeded and sliced
$^1/_2$oz (15g) wholemeal flour
1 pint (575ml) beef stock
pinch dried herbs
1 large can (15oz/425g) red kidney beans

1.   Fry the beef in the cooking oil. Add the sliced onion and green pepper and fry until golden brown.
2.   Add the flour, stirring all the time. Gradually pour on the stock and herbs. Cover and simmer, stirring occasionally, for 2 hours.
3.   Add the beans 15 minutes before the end of the cooking time. Serve with 'free' vegetables.

AUBERGINE CASSEROLE

Serves: 4
Calories per serving: 230

*Measure out the oil carefully in this recipe, as the aubergine
slices soak it up like a sponge!*

2 medium aubergines
$1^1/_2$ tsp salt
2 tbsp corn or olive oil
4 small courgettes, washed, trimmed and thinly sliced
2 medium onions, sliced
2 garlic cloves, crushed
8oz (225g) can chopped tomatoes
$^1/_2$ tsp cayenne pepper
1 tsp ground cumin
1 large can (15oz/425g) chick peas, drained

1.   Peel aubergines and dice flesh, place pieces in a
colander and sprinkle with 1 tsp salt, leave for 30 minutes.
Drain on kitchen paper.
2.   Heat half the oil in a non-stick pan and add chopped
aubergine. Cook for 10 minutes until pieces are evenly
browned on all sides. Drain well on kitchen paper and
transfer with any cooking liquid to a large mixing bowl.
3.   Heat remaining oil, and add onions and garlic to the
pan and cook for 5–7 minutes until onions are soft but not
brown.
4.   Add tomatoes, courgettes, rest of salt, cayenne pepper and cumin and stir well to mix. Cook for 3 minutes
then add to the aubergine mixture.
5.   Stir in the chick peas. Transfer mixture to an ovenproof casserole and bake in a moderate oven until all
vegetables are tender.

CURRY CREOLE

Serves: 4
Calories per serving: 270

Why go out for a curry, when you can cook this up at home?

2 tbsp oil
2 medium onions, thinly sliced
1 garlic clove, crushed
1 green chilli, de-seeded and sliced
4 small courgettes, trimmed and cut into $^1/_4$-in slices
1 large red pepper, de-seeded and sliced
3 tomatoes, blanched, peeled and chopped
2oz (50g) canned pineapple chunks, drained
1 tsp ground coriander
$^1/_2$ tsp each ground cardamon, fenugreek and tumeric
$^1/_4$ tsp hot chilli powder
3 tbsp water
$^1/_2$ pint (275ml) vegetable stock
2 medium bananas, sliced
1-inch slice of creamed coconut

1.   Heat the oil in a large saucepan over moderate heat, then add onions, garlic, chilli, courgettes and red pepper. Cook, stirring occasionally for 10 minutes.
2.   Add tomatoes and pineapple and cook, stirring frequently, for 3 minutes. Combine spices with water in a small bowl to make a smooth paste. Stir into the fruit and vegetable mixture, then pour in the vegetable stock. Increase heat to high and bring stock to the boil. Reduce heat to low, cover and simmer for 15 minutes or until vegetables are cooked. Add bananas.
3.   Stir in creamed coconut, mixing until it dissolves and the liquid thickens. Simmer for further 2 minutes, then transfer to a warmed dish and serve immediately.

CRUNCHY WHOLEWHEAT LASAGNE

Serves: 6
Calories per serving: 360

Delicious and filling, this is a great choice for a Saturday family lunch, with dry white wine, crusty bread and plenty of green salad.

8oz (225g) lean minced meat
10oz (283g) can/jar Italian tomato sauce
$^1/_4$ pint (150ml) beef stock
3oz (75g) Gold low-fat spread
2oz (50g) flour
1 pint (575ml) skimmed milk
1 bay leaf
salt and pepper
8oz (227g) Shape cottage cheese
6oz (175g) wholewheat lasagne, cooked
1oz (25g) fresh wholemeal breadcrumbs
3 tbsp fresh parsley, chopped

1.   Cook the mince until well browned and drain off fat. Stir in the tomato sauce and stock. Cook gently for 3–4 minutes.
2.   Make a sauce by melting the Gold spread and stirring in the flour. Add the skimmed milk and bay leaf. Bring to the boil, stirring continuously until thickened. Remove the bay leaf, season and stir in the cottage cheese.
3.   Cover the base of an ovenproof dish with half the mince and layer with the lasagne and white sauce finishing with a topping of white sauce.
4.   Mix the breadcrumbs and parsley together and sprinkle on top. Bake for 40–45 minutes until bubbling and golden.

SLIMMERS' VEGETABLE BROTH

Serves: 6
Calories per serving: 140

Make up lots of this delicious soup and freeze it for later use. It is absolutely scrumptious and very filling indeed. An ideal choice for lunch, with a crusty roll and some low-fat cheese.

4oz (100g) onions, chopped
6oz (175g) carrots, peeled and sliced
12oz (350g) swede, peeled and diced
4oz (100g) kohl rabi, peeled and diced
4oz (100g) parsnips, peeled and diced
3 cloves garlic, peeled and crushed
2 pints (1 litre) water
1 tbsp tomato purée
salt and pepper
1½tsp oregano
1 tsp thyme
3oz (75g) wholemeal macaroni
8oz (227g) Shape cottage cheese
1 tbsp fresh parsley, chopped

1.   Place all the vegetables in a large saucepan and add the water, tomato purée, seasonings and herbs. Cover and simmer for 30 minutes until tender.
2.   Add the macaroni and cook for a further 10 minutes. Add the cheese and stir into the soup with the parsley. Heat for a few minutes before serving with wholemeal rolls.

BAKED SOLE TARTARE

Serves: 1
Calories per serving: 390

Using sole, this could be a smart starter for a dinner party.
If you choose a cheaper white fish, like cod or coley, this is
inexpensive enough for a family meal.

1 small (4oz/200g) sole (or other white fish) cleaned and
skinned
5fl oz (150ml) water
1 bay leaf
3 peppercorns
5oz (150g) natural yogurt
1 egg
1 tsp capers, chopped
1 gherkin, chopped
grated zest of 1 lemon
1 tbsp parsley, chopped
salt and freshly ground black pepper

1.   Heat oven to 180°C, 350°F, gas mark 4. Place fish in a
shallow pan and add water, bay leaf and peppercorns.
Bring to the boil slowly, cover and poach for 5 minutes.
Drain, place in a shallow ovenproof dish.
2.   Beat together the yogurt and egg mixture with the
remaining ingredients. Spoon the mixture over the fish,
cover and bake for 25 minutes. Serve immediately.

SPANISH PORK

Serves: 6
Calories per serving: 300

Pork isn't as high in calories as most people think – around 40 calories an ounce – so long as you cut off all fat. This recipe uses lean pork fillet or tenderloin and tastes delicious with a selection of 'free' vegetables.

2lb (900g) pork fillet or tenderloin
7oz (200g) onion
1 tbsp olive oil
1 clove garlic
1 red pepper
$^3/_4$ pt (425ml) sieved tomatoes (passata)
8fl oz (225ml) red wine
4fl oz (100ml) water
1 tsp Hermesetas Sprinkle Sweet
8oz (225g) button mushrooms
2oz (50g) green olives
6oz (175g) frozen petits pois
Salt and black pepper

1.   Discard any fat or sinew from the pork and cut into fairly thick slices.
2.   Chop the onion and cook in the oil until soft and golden. Crush the garlic, and deseed the pepper and chop the flesh. Add the garlic, pepper, passata, red wine and water to the pan. Simmer, uncovered, for 15 minutes.
3.   Arrange the pork in a wide-based, shallow dish and pour the sauce over. Cover, and cook at 350°F, 180°C, gas mark 4 for 30 minutes.
4.   Mix in the Sprinkle Sweet, mushrooms, olives and petits pois. Cover again and cook for a further 30 minutes or until the pork is tender. Season to taste.

VALERIE'S VEGETABLE HOT POT

Serves: 4
Calories per serving: 280

This dish was invented by one of our slimmers, Valerie Wyatt. She says 'You can really use any vegetables at all, although I like it with the ones given in the recipe.'

12 small carrots, scraped and sliced
$^1/_2$ aubergine, unpeeled but sliced
8oz (225g) canned small white onions
$^1/_2$ small cabbage, shredded
1 small cauliflower, broken into florets
$^1/_2$ head celery, diced
5 small tomatoes, quartered
1lb (450g) potatoes, peeled and thinly sliced
2 onions, thinly sliced
2 cloves garlic, crushed
2oz (50g) low-fat spread
15fl oz (425ml) hot water
Coleman's Casserole Mix
salt and pepper

1.   Heat oven to 170°C, 325°F, gas mark 3.
2.   Place all the vegetables except the sliced onions and garlic in layers in a large casserole dish, with the sliced potatoes between each layer.
3.   Cook the onion and garlic in the low-fat spread until golden. Mix the casserole mix with the water and add to the onion mixture. Pour over the vegetables. Bake for $1^1/_2$ hours or until tender.

VEGETABLES
LEEKS WITH PIQUANT YOGURT SAUCE

Serves: 4
Calories per serving: 80

They grow sensational leeks up in the North of England, which is why I have included two recipes. In this one, you could use celery or even broccoli as your basic vegetable with the delicious sauce.

4 leeks
5oz (150g) natural low-fat yogurt
2 egg yolks
2 tsp lemon juice
salt and pepper
2 tsp French mustard

1.   Trim leeks, then partially slit them down their length and clean in running water to remove all soil. Put into boiling, salted water and cook gently for 15–20 minutes until soft. Drain well and chill.
2.   Beat yogurt, egg yolks and lemon juice together in a double boiler or in a bowl over hot water. Cook gently until thickened. Season to taste, stir in mustard and allow to cook.
3.   Serve leeks sliced diagonally and topped with the sauce.

BRAISED LEEKS

Serves: 4
Calories per serving: 115

You could try this recipe using whole chicory, celery or cabbage instead of leeks. Chicken or vegetable stock is best and make sure the vegetables are cooked but are still firm with bite-appeal.

12 leeks
1oz (25g) low-fat spread
$^1/_2$ pint (275ml) stock
1 bay leaf
1 peppercorn
salt to taste
2 tsp cornflour

1.   Trim leeks, then partially slit them down their length and clean in running water to remove all soil. Melt the low-fat spread in a shallow oven proof dish and place the leeks on top. Cover with the stock, bay leaf, salt and peppercorns. Cook in the oven at 350°F, 180°C, gas mark 5 until tender, basting from time to time.
2.   When cooked transfer leeks to a warm serving dish and put the stock in a saucepan, discarding the bay leaf and peppercorn. Blend the cornflour with a little cold water, and add to the stock. Bring to the boil, stirring continually. Boil for 1 minute. Pour over the leeks to serve.

SWEET AND SOUR CABBAGE

Serves: 6
Calories per serving: 8

Give an old favourite a new, exciting taste with this recipe. The Hermesetas Sprinkle Sweet contains only 2 calories for each spoonful and the teaspoon of oil contains just 40 calories. The recipe serves 6, so you can eat this dish as one of your 'free' vegetables with a clear conscience!

1 white cabbage, cored and shredded
1 tsp sunflower oil
2 tbsp water
2 tbsp vinegar
2 tsp Hermesetas Sprinkle Sweet
pinch of mixed spice
$^1/_4$ tsp salt

1.   Put the cabbage in a large pan with the rest of the ingredients. Cover and cook over a low heat for 15–20 minutes or until the cabbage is just tender but still crisp. Shake the pan often to prevent sticking.
2.   Just before serving, uncover the pan and cook quickly until all the liquid has evaporated.

SPICED CARROT AND SWEDE

Serves: 6
Calories per serving: 55

Orange juice, ginger and nutmeg spice up two everyday vegetables. Again, you are adding very few calories to the basic 'free' vegetable list (swede contains just 5 calories an ounce), so you can eat plenty of this delicious and filling dish on your Fatfield diet.

4 large carrots, peeled and sliced
1lb (450g) swede, peeled and sliced
1 tsp sunflower oil
juice and grated zest of 1 orange
pinch each of ground ginger and nutmeg

1. Place carrots and swede in a shallow ovenproof dish. Combine the rest of the ingredients, and pour over.
2. Lightly cover with foil and bake in a hot oven, 190°C, 375°F, gas mark 5, for about 45 minutes or until tender.

DRESSINGS
SPICY TOMATO SAUCE

Serves: 4
Calories per serving: 15

Delicious with grilled or roast chicken, fish or kebabs, this is a recipe you can make in quantity. To add bulk, include a few pulped canned tomatoes (from your 'free' vegetable list).

8fl oz (225ml) tomato juice
2fl oz (50ml) wine vinegar
1 tsp Worcestershire sauce
2oz (50g) onion, finely chopped
1 tsp dry basil
salt and freshly ground black pepper
1 tsp lemon juice
pinch of Hermesetas Sprinkle Sweet
chopped parsley to garnish

Place all the ingredients except garnish in a saucepan and bring to the boil, cover and simmer for $^1/_2$ hour or until the sauce has thickened. Serve hot or cold.

BASIC SALAD DRESSING

Serves: 4
Calories per serving: 2

3 tbsp cider vinegar
2 tbsp lemon juice
grated rind of $^1/_2$ lemon
1 tsp mixed herbs and 1 clove garlic, crushed
1 tsp french mustard
salt and pepper

Mix all the ingredients in a blender or screw top jar.

BARBECUE SAUCE

Serves: 6
Calories per serving: 65

This is a 'must' for those summer barbecues and al fresco *suppers.*

$^1/_2$oz (15g) butter
1 tbsp sunflower oil
1 clove garlic, crushed
1 small onion, chopped
4 tbsp tomato ketchup
1 tbsp brown fruity sauce
1 tbsp Worcestershire sauce
1 tbsp soya sauce
1 tsp French mustard
salt and pepper
6 fl oz (175ml) hot water
$^1/_2$ beef stock cube
6oz (175g) tomatoes
2 tsp Hermesetas Sprinkle Sweet

1. Melt butter in a small pan with the oil. Add the garlic and onion and cook until soft and translucent.
2. Stir in the tomato ketchup, brown sauce, Worcestershire sauce, soya sauce and mustard. Season lightly with salt and pepper. Dissolve the stock cube in the water and add to the pan. Cover and simmer for 10 minutes.
3. Peel the tomatoes, cut in half and discard the seeds and juice. Chop the flesh and add to the pan. Simmer uncovered for 5 minutes. Purée in a blender or processor. Add the Hermesetas Sprinkle Sweet and reheat, do not boil. Serve with barbecued or grilled meat or fish.

DESSERTS
TONI'S AMAZING TRIFLE

Serves: 4
Calories per serving: 90

Toni Tompsett, my assistant, is a slimmer with a young family to feed. This recipe satisfies her own sweet tooth and theirs!

1 Bird's Strawberry Sugar Free Jelly
8oz (225g) fresh or frozen strawberries
4 sponge fingers
$1/_2$ pint (275ml) skimmed milk
1 tbsp custard powder
Hermesetas Sprinkle Sweet to taste
4 heaped tbsp Anchor Light aerosol cream

1.   Break the sponge fingers into four individual bowls. Add 2oz (50g) strawberries to each, cover with $1/_4$ of the dissolved jelly. Leave the jelly to set.
2.   Mix the custard powder with 1 tbsp of cold milk. Bring the remaining milk to the boil and then pour onto the custard mixture stirring all the time. Off the heat add sweetener to taste. Leave to cool, then pour over the jelly. Add a swirl of Anchor Light aerosol cream just before serving.

APRICOT AND ORANGE MOUSSE

Serves: 6
Calories per serving: 105

This is packed with goodies, and absolutely scrumptious.
Make it in advance for a special occasion or a dinner party.
You can keep it in the fridge for 24 hours before serving.

5oz (150g) ready-to-eat dried apricots
2 fl oz (50ml) water
7 fl oz (200ml) orange juice
1 envelope powdered gelatine
3 tbsp Hermesetas Sprinkle Sweet
7.7oz (215g) low-fat evaporated milk, chilled
1 egg white
orange peel to decorate

1.   Place the apricots in a saucepan, add the water and $^3/_4$ of the orange juice. Cover and cook until tender, about 15–20 minutes. Turn into a basin and allow to cool.
2.   Sprinkle the gelatine onto the remaining orange juice in a small basin and leave to soak for 10 minutes. Then stand the basin in a pan of simmering water until the gelatine has dissolved.
3.   Purée the apricots and their cooking liquid in a blender or food processor. Add the dissolved gelatine and Hermesetas Sprinkle Sweet and mix well.
4.   Whisk the evaporated milk until thick and foamy. Whisk the egg white until stiff. Fold the evaporated milk and egg white into the apricot mixture and then divide between 6 dishes, chill until set. Decorate with grated orange peel.

NECTARINES IN PEACH SAUCE

Serves: 6
Calories per serving: 140

This is a wonderful, fruity, boozy, posh-looking summer pud. Serve it with fromage frais or yogurt for a dinner party or special Sunday lunch and wait for the compliments!

1 large can (15oz/425g) peaches in juice
6 nectarines
Strip of thinly pared orange peel
3oz (75g) blackcurrants, fresh or frozen
2 tbsp unsweetened apple juice
2 tbsp Hermesetas Sprinkle Sweet
1 tbsp Cassis
2 tbsp Cointreau or Grand Marnier

1.   Drain the peaches and place the juice in a large pan with the nectarines and orange rind in a single layer. Add enough water to just cover the fruit. Bring to the boil slowly. Cover and simmer gently for 10 minutes. Leave to cool in the juice.
2.   Meanwhile, cook the blackcurrants in the apple juice in a small covered pan until tender. Rub through a sieve and mix with 1 tbsp Sprinkle Sweet and the Cassis.
3.   Purée the drained peaches with the orange liqueur and remaining Sprinkle Sweet.
4.   'Marble' the two fruit purées on a serving dish.
5.   Peel the nectarines and serve on the sauce.

FRUIT BRULÉE

Serves: 4
Calories per serving: 230

You can prepare this in advance and add the finishing touches before it is placed under the grill. Let your guests chat among themselves while you watch it carefully.

4oz (100g) strawberries, halved
4oz (100g) raspberries
2 tbsp blackcurrant liqueur
5fl oz (150ml) whipping cream
5fl oz (150ml) Greek yogurt
1oz (25g) golden granulated sugar

1. Mix the fruit with the liqueur in an ovenproof dish.
2. Whip the cream until it forms soft peaks, then carefully fold in the yogurt. Spoon the mixture over the fruit and smooth the surface. Cover and chill for 1 hour.
3. Sprinkle the sugar over the top. Flash under the grill until golden. Serve immediately or chill in the fridge until the topping is hard and crunchy.

JAMAICAN BANANAS

Serves: 4
Calories per serving: 115

This recipe will make you feel as though you're basking on a terrace under the stars in the West Indies. Savour every spoonful slowly, for a sensual experience.

4 medium bananas, peeled
1 tbsp Hermesetas Sprinkle Sweet
$^1/_2$ tsp ground cinnamon
4 tbsp Bacardi
$^1/_2$ tsp lemon zest, finely grated
zest of $^1/_2$ a small orange, finely grated

1. Place each banana on a piece of foil. Cover with Sprinkle Sweet and then the cinnamon. Pour 1 tbsp Bacardi on each banana, and wrap in the foil so no juice can escape.
2. Bake in a moderate oven or on a barbecue for 5 minutes. Open and sprinkle with the zest.

CHAPTER ELEVEN

BREAKFASTS
IN A HURRY

No time for breakfast? On the Fatfield Diet, you should definitely *make* time for an early morning meal. But, you certainly don't have to spend hours slaving over a hot stove, or get up at dawn. In fact, if you truly can't face eating before you leave home to go to work, you can pack up your breakfast and take it with you.

Traditionally, we tend to eat either a sketchy snack of cereals or toast, or a huge, cooked breakfast. The first is certainly better than nothing, but the second can be packed with fat and calories and hardly ideal for slimmers.

Here's a selection of recipes which provide a tasty, appetizing start to the day, for a very small number of calories. The cooked dishes are so quick to prepare that you can serve them up in less than 10 minutes. The cold meals can be prepared the night before, or placed in an airtight container to pack into your shopping bag or briefcase. If you are really rushed, a blender is a useful gadget for whizzing up quick, nourishing breakfasts with yogurt, fruit and juices. Storecupboard breakfast basics include muesli, bran and yogurt.

On the Continent, cheese and meat are breakfast basics – both can be tasty so long as they are combined with something refreshing such as citrus fruit or tomatoes, and you don't overdo the portion sizes.

Although we don't usually think of serving salad greens

179

at breakfast time, it is worth keeping some washed watercress in the fridge to add a spot of colour and extra iron to your breakfast meal.

In this chapter all the recipes are for one person only, as in most households people tend to 'do their own' thing at breakfast time.

CHEESEY TOMATOES ON TOAST

Serves: 1
Calories per serving: 250

2 slices wholemeal toast
2 large tomatoes, sliced
4 tbsp cottage cheese
Watercress to garnish

1.   Toast one side of each slice of wholemeal bread under the grill.
2.   Transfer to an ovenproof dish, untoasted side up. Place the sliced tomatoes on top of the bread. Return to the grill until the tomatoes are soft.
3.   Place 2 tablespoons cottage cheese on top of each slice, and garnish with watercress. I like this with loads of Worcestershire sauce!

SWEETCORN GRILL

Serves: 1
Calories per serving: 235

3oz (75g) canned sweetcorn, drained
1oz (25g) low-fat Cheddar cheese
1 slice wholemeal toast
1 tomato, thinly sliced

1.   Heat the corn and cheese gently in a small saucepan until the cheese melts.
2.   Place on the bread, cover with the slices of tomato and grill until the tomato is cooked.

LIQUID BREAKFAST

Serves: 1
Calories per serving: 160

For a more substantial breakfast that's packed with goodness, pour your drink over a 1oz (25g) portion of any unsweetened cereal and top with chopped fresh fruit. Recommended as a Saturday morning breakfast for footballers or hockey players.

1 small carton (5oz/150g) natural, low-fat yogurt
1 small banana
1 tbsp wheatgerm
2 tbsp unsweetened orange juice
Pinch of cinnamon

1.   Whizz up everything together in a blender, and drink slowly.

SCRAMBLED EGGS WITH MUSHROOMS

Serves: 1
Calories per serving: 235

Mushrooms taste better, look plumper and go further if they are poached in water instead of fried. What's more they only 'cost' 4 calories per 1oz (25g), instead of 50!

2 eggs
2 tbsp skimmed milk
Salt and black pepper
3oz (75g) button mushrooms
Watercress to garnish
2 crispbreads

1.   Beat together the eggs, skimmed milk and season to taste.
2.   Cook over a low heat, stirring all the time or microwave, stirring twice until creamy but *not* overcooked.
3.   Meanwhile, poach the mushrooms whole in a little water for 5 minutes.
4.   Serve the scrambled eggs and mushrooms on a plate with the crispbreads and garnish with watercress.

BUMPER BACON ROLL

Serves: 1
Calories per serving: 310

1 large bap or crispy roll
2oz (50g) streaky bacon
2 tomatoes
Watercress
1oz (25g) sweetcorn

1. Split open the bap or roll.
2. Grill the bacon on a rack until crisp, discarding any fat.
3. Halve the tomatoes and grill, cut side up.
4. Sandwich everything together, adding watercress and sweetcorn. It will be oozy, but delicious!

MELON AND MUESLI FRUIT BASKET

Serves: 1
Calories per serving: 250

½ small Ogen or honeydew melon
1oz (25g) unsweetened muesli
1 red apple, cored and chopped
½ small carton low-fat fruit-flavoured yogurt
A few seedless grapes, chopped
Cinnamon

1. Remove the seeds from the melon. Remove the flesh with a teaspoon making 'ball' shapes or use a melon baller if you have one.
2. Mix the melon flesh with the muesli and chopped apple, and pile back into the shell.
3. Top with the yogurt, chopped grapes and a sprinkling of cinnamon.

BOSTON BAKED BEANS

Serves: 1
Calories per serving: 340

1 small can (5.3oz/150g) baked beans
1 tsp Dijon mustard
1 small can (7oz/200g) tomatoes
2 rashers streaky bacon, grilled on a rack
2 crispbreads

1. Heat the baked beans in a small pan.
2. Add the mustard and tomatoes and heat through.
3. Serve in a bowl with the bacon crumbled on top, and the crispbreads for dunking.

GRAPE AND LEMON CHEESE PITTA

Serves: 1
Calories per serving: 300

Wholemeal pitta bread is super for transporting a scrumptious breakfast to work. Each piece contains just 165 calories – stuff it with a rasher of crispy grilled streaky bacon, sliced tomatoes, lettuce and add an apple for another great early morning meal which 'costs' under 300 calories.

1 pitta bread, split
2oz (50g) Shape Low Fat Soft Cheese
Squeeze of lemon juice
10 seedless grapes

1. Make a pocket along the length of the pitta bread.
2. Mix together the cheese, lemon juice and grapes in a small bowl.
3. Stuff the mixture into the pitta bread. Yum.

FISHERMAN'S BREAKFAST

Serves: 1
Calories per serving: 225

1 Bird's Eye fish cake
2 tomatoes, halved
1 dsp tartare sauce
1 tbsp natural, low-fat yogurt
Lettuce, cucumber and watercress
1 slice wholemeal toast
Slice of lemon to garnish

1. Grill the fish cake on both sides until crisp.
2. Grill the tomatoes on a rack, cut side up.
3. Mix together the tartare sauce and yogurt.
4. Place lettuce, cucumber and watercress on a plate and top with the slice of toast and fish cake.
5. Pour the sauce on top and garnish with a slice of lemon.

FRUITY BREAKFAST ROLL

Serves: 1
Calories per serving: 205

1 crusty wholemeal roll
1 apple, cored and chopped
½oz (15g) raisins
1 tbsp lemon juice
1 tbsp cottage cheese or low-fat fromage frais

1. Split the roll.
2. Mix the remaining ingredients together.
3. Pile on to one half of the roll, and place the second half on top.

BLACKBERRY AND APPLE SUNDAE

Serves: 1
Calories per serving: 200

1oz (25g) bran cereal
1 medium apple, cored and chopped
½ small carton low-fat blackcurrant or raspberry yogurt
A few blackberries to garnish

1. Place the cereal in the bottom of a large sundae glass.
2. Mix in the chopped apple.
3. Pour yogurt over the top.
4. Garnish with blackberries.

BANANA SANDWICH WITH HONEY AND YOGURT

Serves: 1
Calories per serving: 260

1 medium banana
2 medium slices wholemeal bread
2 tbsp natural, low-fat yogurt
1 tsp runny honey

1. Slice the banana and place on one piece of bread.
2. Pour over the yogurt, and drizzle honey on top.
3. Place the second slice of bread on top, cut the sandwich in half and serve.

CHAPTER TWELVE

PACKED LUNCHES, SNACKS AND NAUGHTY NIBBLES

If you really want to take control of your weight, you must never get caught short without the right kind of snack food. Fast food joints are everywhere – and they're just waiting for slimmers with rumbling tums to wander in. On the Fatfield diet, you eat so much – including between-meals snacks – that you should never be hungry. So, make sure that you have a good stock of fruit, salad vegetables, and low-calorie supermarket goodies like slimmer's fromage frais, yogurt, and soups. Work out when your danger times are, and be prepared. For instance, if you're always ravenous when you get home from work and start preparing the evening meal, nibble a low-calorie snack then, to stave off the hunger pangs.

It's always a good idea to take a packed lunch to work. That way, you won't be tempted by canteen chips. In this chapter, there's a really super selection of interesting packed meals. Invest in a set of good airtight containers and a small vacuum flask, and add pretty paper napkins, so your midday break becomes a feast.

Late-night telly watching often brings on an attack of the naughty nibbles, particularly if you are watching a food or drink commercial. The answer is to whizz up a treat from our suggestions, rather than digging into the biscuit tin.

PASTA SALAD

Serves: 1
Calories per serving: 180

You can use any leftovers such as chicken, green beans, tuna, broccoli or melon balls with this easy salad. If you add a crusty wholemeal roll, and follow with a piece of fresh fruit, you'll have a satisfying lunch at around 350 calories.

2oz (50g) cooked pasta twists, cooled
1oz (25g) Edam cheese, cut into ½in (1cm) cubes
½ small green pepper, cored, deseeded and sliced
½ small red pepper, cored, deseeded and sliced
1 tbsp low-fat fromage frais
Curry powder to taste

1. Mix the pasta, cheese and slices of pepper in a bowl.
2. To make the dressing blend the fromage frais with curry powder to taste.
3. Combine the dressing with the pasta salad.

LEMON DIP WITH FRUIT CRUDITÉS

Serves: 4
Calories per serving: About 200

4oz (100g) Edam cheese, grated finely
2 tbsp boiling water
6oz (175g) low-fat fromage frais
Juice and grated rind of ½ small lemon
¼ tsp ground ginger
Fruit crudités
1 large green and 1 large red apple, cored and cut into
   segments, dipped in lemon juice
A few grapes, pineapple chunks (canned in juice), sliced
   kiwi fruit or mango

1. Place the grated Edam in a bowl, add the boiling water
and stir.
2. Add the fromage frais, lemon juice and rind and
ground ginger to make a dip.
3. Spoon the dip into a glass dish and chill for 30 minutes.
4. Arrange the fruit crudités decoratively on a serving
plate, with the dip in the centre. For a packed lunch, put ¼
of the dip in a small airtight container, and pack a selection
of fruit separately.

CHICKEN AND VEGETABLE SALAD

Serves: 2
Calories per serving: 215

½ small cauliflower
4oz (100g) carrots, sliced thinly
4oz (100g) frozen green beans
2oz (50g) frozen peas
4oz (100g) canned sweetcorn
1 celery stick, chopped finely
4oz (100g) cooked chicken, skin removed and diced
Chopped parsley to garnish
Dressing
4 tbsp natural, low-fat yogurt
½ tsp horseradish sauce
½ tsp lemon juice

1. Break the cauliflower into florets.
2. Cook the cauliflower, carrots, beans and peas in boiling salted water for 5 minutes. Drain.
3. Mix all the vegetables and the diced chicken together in a bowl.
4. Mix together the dressing ingredients and pour over the salad. Toss well, garnish with parsley and serve, or pack in an airtight container.

TOMATO, CARROT AND ONION SOUP

Serves: 2
Calories per serving: 90

Use canned chopped tomatoes as a base for other filling soups. Just add leftover vegetables, chopped finely, or even a few leftover prawns or strips of ham. This particular recipe also tastes great chilled and travels well in a wide-necked vacuum flask (take the yogurt separately and eat the rest with a chopped apple as your pud!).

1 large can (14oz/397g) chopped tomatoes
2 large carrots, grated
1 small onion, chopped finely
½pt (275ml) chicken stock
1 tsp dried basil
Pinch of nutmeg
Salt and black pepper
2 tbsp natural, low-fat yogurt
Chopped parsley to garnish

1. Place the tomatoes in a large saucepan.
2. Add the carrot, onion, stock, basil and a pinch of nutmeg.
3. Bring to the boil, stirring, cover and simmer for 20 minutes. Check the seasoning – add just a touch of salt and ground black pepper if necessary.
4. Serve with a swirl of yogurt and a sprinkling of parsley on top.

TANGY HAM ON TOAST

Serves: 1
Calories per serving: 210

This is a scrummy lunch for one person. Pile on plenty of 'free' salad vegetables (page 35), and have a juicy peach or pear afterwards.

1 slice wholemeal bread
½ apple, cored and sliced
1oz (25g) lean ham
1 dsp tomato chutney
1 pickled onion, chopped
1oz (25g) grated low-fat Cheddar cheese
Parsley, lettuce, cucumber and watercress to garnish

1.   Toast the bread on both sides.
2.   Arrange the apple slices, then the ham on top of the toast.
3.   Spread the tomato chutney over the ham and sprinkle with onion.
4.   Sprinkle with the grated cheese and place under a hot grill until the cheese is bubbly.
5.   Serve sprinkled with chopped parsley and garnished with salad greens.

COTTAGE BAKED POTATO WITH MINTY TOMATO SALAD

Serves: 1
Calories per serving: 255

1 7oz (200g) baking potato, scrubbed and pricked
2 large tomatoes, sliced
2oz (50g) cottage cheese with chives
Dressing
1 tsp mint sauce
1 dsp wine vinegar

1.   Bake the potato in a moderate oven (400°F, 200°C, gas mark 6), or cook in a microwave oven until cooked through.
2.   Meanwhile, place the sliced tomatoes on a plate, mix together the dressing ingredients and pour on top. Chill the salad until required.
3.   Split the potato, spoon over the cottage cheese, and serve with the salad.

FANTASTIC FATFIELD FILLINGS

Fed up with stuffing your sandwiches, baps and rolls with the same old low-calorie fillings? Here are six mouthwatering ideas, calorie counted. Add an extra 100 calories for your bap or roll, 165 calories if you pop the filling into a warmed wholemeal pitta, or 140 if you use two slices of wholemeal bread to make a sandwich. Don't forget to add plenty of 'free' salad vegetables from the list on page 35, and fresh fruit or a low-fat yogurt for dessert.

1. 2oz (50g) cooked, sliced chicken (no skin), mixed with 2 chopped radishes, diced cucumber and tossed in dressing made from 1 tablespoon reduced-calorie mayonnaise and ½ level teaspoon horseradish sauce. *Calories: 135.*

2. 2oz (50g) low-fat soft cheese mixed with ½oz (15g) raisins, grated carrot, chopped celery and lemon juice. *Calories: 135.*

3. 3oz (75g) baked beans with chopped onion, 1 dessertspoon sweet pickle, 1 teaspoon Dijon mustard and ½oz (15g) grated low-fat Cheddar cheese. *Calories: 120.*

4. 1 pear, cored and sliced, lemon juice, ½oz (15g) chopped lean ham, 1 tablespoon cottage cheese and sprigs of fresh mint. *Calories: 90.*

5. 2 sardines, drained and mashed with lemon juice and 1 tablespoon natural, low-fat yogurt, then mixed with diced cucumber, red and green peppers, cored, deseeded and diced, and freshly ground black pepper. *Calories: 135.*

6. 1 small banana, sliced, mixed with 1 sliced, drained apricot half (canned in juice), lemon juice, ½oz (15g) raisins, 1 dessertspoon low-fat fromage frais and a pinch of grated nutmeg. *Calories: 105.*

CHEAP AND CHEESEY LUNCHES

Our Fatfield slimmers are a hard-working bunch, with many of the women holding down several jobs as well as looking after a family. It's all too tempting to skip meals, but that is a certain way to diet disaster. Here are some quick cheesey lunchtime ideas from Fatfield slimmers Sheila Turnbull and Ann McKenna.

1.   *Tuna Bake:* Drain a 3½oz (99g) can of tuna in brine and place in an ovenproof dish. Heat 1 can (7½oz/213g) creamed mushrooms and pour on top of the tuna. Mix 2oz (50g) grated low-fat cheese with 2oz (50g) wholemeal breadcrumbs and sprinkle on top. Bake in a moderate oven (350°F, 180°C, gas mark 4) for 10 minutes, then flash under the grill until golden. *Serves 2. Calories per serving: 290.*

2.   *Cheese and Apple Toasts:* Toast one side of a slice of wholemeal bread. Spread the other side with ½ teaspoon French mustard. Peel and thinly slice 1 apple. Place the slices on top of the mustard, squeeze lemon juice on top and top with 1oz (25g) grated Edam cheese. Place under the grill until the cheese melts. *Serves 1. Calories per serving: 215.*

3.   *Cheesey Fish Snack:* Toast one side of a slice of wholemeal bread, and cover the other side with 2oz (50g) cooked smoked cod or haddock and sliced onion. Sprinkle with salt and freshly ground black pepper and 1oz (25g) grated low-fat Cheddar cheese. Grill under a moderate heat to allow the fish to heat through and the cheese to go golden brown. *Serves 1. Calories per serving: 210.*

TELLY NIBBLES

Here are six ideas for sweet or savoury nibbles and drinks. They are for those awful moments when you feel you must have something – or dive into the biscuit tin! They're all very low in calories and very satisfying.

1. 2 Ryvitas, topped with sliced tomato, cucumber and 2 tablespoons Shape coleslaw, and a mug of Oxo to drink. *Calories: 100.*

2. 1 slice wholemeal bread spread with 1 tablespoon Shape Fromage Frais and a mug of Ovaltine Options to drink. *Calories: 120.*

3. Huge mixed salad topped with sliced pear and 2 tablespoons cottage cheese, washed down with a glass of low-alcohol wine. *Calories: 135.*

4. 1 mug Batchelor's Slim-A-Soup with wholemeal toast croûtons and ½oz (15g) grated Edam cheese on top. *Calories: 115.*

5. 1 carton Shape Fromage Frais mixed with 1 chopped banana and a sprinkling of muesli, and lemon tea to drink. *Calories: 180.*

5. Open sandwich of 1 slice of slimmer's bread, lettuce, watercress, sliced orange, 2 dates and 1 tablespoon natural low-fat yogurt, and a mug of Bovril to drink. *Calories: 120.*

FATFIELD SALAD DRESSINGS

These are all extra low in calories, and very tasty indeed. Try them, and experiment with your own no-fat versions.

1. *Yogurt and Lemon:* Mix together a 5oz (150g) carton natural, low-fat yogurt, 2 tbsp lemon juice, 2 tsp chopped fresh herbs such as basil, mint or fennel leaves to taste or ½ tsp dried herbs and freshly ground black pepper. Chill for 1 hour before serving. *Serves 4. Calories per serving: 20.*

2. *Orange or Lemon Vinaigrette:* Shake together in a screw-topped jar, 3 tbsp wine vinegar, 1 tbsp fresh orange or lemon juice, 1 tbsp grated orange or lemon rind, ½ tsp French mustard and freshly ground black pepper and salt to taste. *Serves 2. Calories per serving: 5.*

3. *Spicy Tomato Juice Dressing:* Shake together in a screw-topped jar 4 tbsp tomato juice, 4 tbsp wine vinegar, 1 tsp Worcestershire sauce, 2 tsp finely chopped shallots or spring onions, ½ teaspoon dried basil, freshly ground black pepper and salt to taste. *Serves 4. Calories per serving: 5.*

FAVOURITE FATFIELD DRINKS

Got a thirst? Don't just reach for a boring old can of low-calorie fizzy drink. Try these instead:

Minimal Calories

1.   *Pink Tonic:* Add a dash of Angostura bitters to a glass of low-calorie tonic water, and garnish with a slice of peach or orange.

2.   *Ginger Kick:* Mix 1 tablespoon low calorie lime juice with 1 glass of low-calorie ginger ale, top up with ice and garnish with a slice of lime or lemon and cucumber slices.

3.   *Pineapple Crush:* Chop up a few bits of leftover pineapple, canned in juice. Pour on the leftover juice, top up with soda and crushed ice.

4.   *Chilled Herbal Teas:* Try making any herbal tea, chilling it, then serving with ice and fresh lemon, orange or grapefruit juice.

Under 100 Calories

1.   *Choccy comforter:* Make up one sachet Ovaltine Options Choc-au-lait and serve with an After Eight Mint for dunking.

2.   *Spritzer:* Pour out a small glass of white wine, and top up your glass with soda, ice and lemon and a sprig of mint.

3.   *Sherry Toddy:* Make up a mug of Bovril and stir in 1 small glass of dry sherry.

CHAPTER THIRTEEN

FAMILY FAVOURITES

The greatest test for any slimmer is sitting down at the table to a big, family meal. For women, it is very hard indeed not to nibble while you're preparing food designed to fill up hungry children and non-slimming men. When the meal finally appears on the table, you really can't be expected to resist tasting it!

On the Fatfield Diet, the family meal is very important indeed. Our slimmers always sit down to a substantial evening meal, and usually serve up exactly the same fare for the family. The subtle differences in the way the dishes are cooked do nothing to impair the taste – they just cut calories and make the meal far healthier, too.

Storecupboard basics for family dishes like these include slimmers' soups (for casseroles and sauces), canned tomatoes, low-fat cheese and natural, low-fat yogurt.

Here are 12 recipes for filling, inexpensive dishes which are all old favourites, with a new, low-calorie twist! Even the Sunday roast is included, plus good old fish and chips!

LIVER, CHIPOLATA AND BEAN CASSEROLE

Serves: 4
Calories per serving: 275

This is the kind of hot, filling supper that it's great to come home to on a winter night, and the calories are so low that you can afford to have a 5oz (150g) baked potato or some noodles to go with it.

4oz (100g) low-fat chipolata sausages
12oz (350g) lamb's liver, sliced thinly
1 onion, sliced
1 can (10.4oz/285g) Weight Watchers from Heinz
    Tomato Soup
2 tsp Worcestershire sauce
1 tsp wine vinegar
1 tsp Dijon mustard
Salt and black pepper
1 medium can (7.9oz/225g) Weight Watchers from Heinz
    Baked Beans
Parsley sprigs to garnish

1.   Grill the sausages on a rack so any fat drips through. When just cooked, cool and cut into 1in (2.5cm) pieces.
2.   Place the liver in an ovenproof casserole with the sausages and onion.
3.   Mix the soup with the Worcestershire sauce, vinegar and mustard.
4.   Season to taste and pour over the liver mixture.
5.   Cover and cook in a moderate oven (350°F, 180°C, gas mark 4) for 45 minutes.
6.   Remove from the oven, and stir in the baked beans. Cook for a further 10 minutes and serve, garnished with parsley sprigs.

BANGERS AND MASH WITH ONION, MUSHROOM AND TOMATO GRAVY

Serves: 4
Calories per serving: 310

Add plenty of green vegetables from your 'free' list (page 35), and finish this substantial meal with a baked apple plus a squirt of aerosol cream. Calorie total? Under 400!

8 low-fat pork sausages
1lb (450g) potatoes, peeled weight
¼pt (150ml) skimmed milk
Salt and black pepper
1 large onion, chopped finely
2oz (50g) button mushrooms, sliced
1 large can (14oz/397g) tomatoes
Pinch of mixed herbs
1 beef stock cube
Parsley sprigs or watercress to garnish

1.   Grill the sausages on a rack, so any fat drips through and can be discarded.
2.   Meanwhile, slice the potatoes, cook until tender and mash with skimmed milk and a little salt and freshly ground black pepper to taste.
3.   To make the gravy place the chopped onion, mushrooms and tomatoes in a pan with the mixed herbs and cook gently for 5 minutes.
4.   Dissolve the stock cube in a little water and juice from the tomatoes, then pour back into the gravy and stir. Simmer gently for 2 minutes.
5.   Serve with the potatoes piled in the centre of an oval dish, and the sausages and gravy arranged around them. Garnish with sprigs of parsley or watercress.

TANGY CHEESEBURGERS AND BEANS

Serves: 4
Calories per serving: 265

Add a bap if you like, for an authentic burger bar meal, plus a mixed salad and 3oz (75g) oven chips. Calorie total: 450.

12oz (350g) lean minced beef
1 onion, chopped
½oz (15g) bread, as breadcrumbs
1 beef stock cube, crumbled
1 tsp mixed herbs
Salt and black pepper
1 egg, beaten
2oz (50g) mushrooms, chopped
2 tsp horseradish sauce
1oz (25g) grated Edam cheese
1 medium can (7.9oz/225g) Weight Watchers from Heinz
   Baked Beans

1.   Put the minced beef, onion, breadcrumbs, crumbled stock cube, herbs and seasoning in a bowl, and mix.
2.   Add the beaten egg, mix well and divide the mixture into 4 flat round cakes.
3.   Place in a heatproof dish and grill for 4–5 minutes on each side under a medium heat until cooked through.
4.   Carefully remove from the dish, and place on kitchen paper to remove any excess fat. Keep hot until ready to serve.
5.   Poach the mushrooms in a little water until soft. Drain, and stir in the horseradish sauce and season to taste. Spoon the mushrooms over each burger, and top with the grated cheese.
6.   Pop back under a high grill until the cheese is melted.
7.   Serve with the heated baked beans.

BEEF STEW WITH NEWCASTLE BROWN ALE

Serves: 4
Calories per serving: 190

Guaranteed to warm a man's heart, this substantial supper dish can be served with rice, a small baked potato or just a salad. It also reheats and freezes well.

1lb (450g) lean chuck steak, cubed
1 medium onion, sliced
1 carrot, sliced
1 clove garlic, crushed
3oz (75g) button mushrooms
½pt (275ml) Newcastle Brown Ale (or use Guinness for a richer gravy)
1 beef stock cube
1 tsp malt vinegar
Pinch of nutmeg
Salt and black pepper
1 bay leaf
Chopped parsley to garnish

1.   Dry fry the steak in a heavy-based, non-stick pan to seal the meat.
2.   Place in a deep casserole with the onion, carrot, garlic and mushrooms.
3.   Blend the ale with the stock cube, vinegar and a pinch of nutmeg. Season to taste.
4.   Pour the ale over the meat and vegetables in the casserole, and add the bay leaf.
5.   Cover, and cook in a moderate oven (325°F, 170°C, gas mark 3) for 1½ hours or until the meat is tender. Discard the bay leaf.
6.   Serve garnished with chopped parsley.

LAMB'S KIDNEYS IN PIQUANT YOGURT SAUCE

Serves: 4
Calories per serving: About 135

Add lots of 'free' vegetables (page 35), and a medium-sized baked potato, and you'll enjoy a vitamin-, mineral- and fibre-packed supper for under 350 calories.

8 lamb's kidneys (about 1lb/450g)
5fl oz (150ml) beef stock
4oz (100g) mushrooms, sliced
1 tbsp tomato purée
2 tsp prepared English mustard
1 small carton (5oz/150g) natural, low-fat yogurt
Salt and black pepper to taste
2 tsp cornflour
1 tbsp chopped parsley to garnish

1. Skin the kidneys, cut them in half and remove the cores. Place in a saucepan with the stock, mushrooms and tomato purée.
2. Cook very gently, covered, for 10 minutes or until tender.
3. Stir in the mustard and yogurt. Season to taste.
4. Mix the cornflour with a little cold water and stir into the pan. Simmer, stirring, for 2–3 minutes.
5. Sprinkle with parsley and serve with salad or vegetables from the 'free' list.

TURKEY ROAST WITH PLUM AND APPLE SAUCE

Serves: 4
Calories per portion: 370

Add piles of 'free' vegetables (page 35) for a tasty, midweek treat. If the family wants roast potatoes, cook them the Fatfield way – parboil peeled potatoes, brush with vegetable oil and place under the grill, turning occasionally, until brown. In this way you can have a 2oz (50g) chunk of roast potato for only 55 calories!

1½lb (675g) parsnips, quartered
1 turkey breast roll roast, about 1¼lb (550g)
4 medium cooking apples, peeled, cored and quartered
4 large plums, stoned and chopped (if you use canned
    plums, wash off all the syrup carefully)
2 tsp Hermesetas Sprinkle Sweet
Watercress to garnish

1.   Parboil the parsnips in boiling salted water for 3 minutes. Drain well.
2.   Spread a large piece of foil over a roasting tin, place the turkey breast on it and surround with the parsnips and half the cooking apples. Seal the foil on top of the meat, and cook in a moderate oven (350°F, 180°C, gas mark 4) for 1½ hours, unwrapping the foil for the last 10 minutes.
3.   Meanwhile, make the sauce: cook the rest of the apples and the plums together in a little water for 15 minutes, or until soft. Add the Sprinkle Sweet. Mash or whirl in the blender if you prefer a smoother sauce.
4.   Serve the sauce in a warmed jug, and the roast garnished with watercress.

LAMB OR PORK KEBABS

Serves: 4
Calories per serving: About 230

Dish these up with the barbecue sauce on page 173 for a midweek treat that's bound to go down well with the whole family. Delicious cherry tomatoes are available at most supermarkets now, and are perfect for kebabs.

1lb (450g) lean, boneless leg of lamb or pork tenderloin
1 large red pepper, cored and deseeded
1 large green pepper, cored and deseeded
4oz (100g) button mushrooms
8oz (225g) cherry tomatoes
A little oil for brushing

1. Cut the meat into cubes, discarding any fat and gristle.
2. Cut the deseeded peppers into squares.
3. Thread the lamb or pork, peppers, mushrooms and tomatoes onto skewers.
4. Brush the vegetables with a little oil.
5. Cook under a preheated grill, turning frequently, until the meat is cooked through and tender.

CHEESE AND CORN BAKE

Serves: 4
Calories per serving: 275

Serve with a crisp green salad.

1lb (450g) potatoes (peeled weight), cooked
1oz (25g) low-fat spread
1 large can (11½oz/326g) sweetcorn, drained
8oz (225g) cottage cheese with chives
4oz (100g) lean unsmoked back bacon, grilled on a rack
and chopped
1 tbsp chopped parsley
Salt and black pepper

1. Boil the potatoes until tender. Drain and mash with
the low-fat spread.
2. Stir the drained sweetcorn, cottage cheese, chopped
bacon and parsley into the mashed potato. Season to taste.
3. Spoon into an ovenproof dish and bake at 400°F,
200°C, gas mark 6 for 20–30 minutes until golden on top.

CHICKEN AND VEGETABLE PIE

Serves: 4
Calories per serving: 380

This basic recipe can be used for fish pie, too. Just leave out the chicken and add cooked, flaked white fish to the vegetables with the peas and seasoning. The calorie count will be slightly lower as white fish has around 25 calories per 1oz (25g), compared with 42 for chicken. If you're really feeling flush, throw in a few prawns (2 calories each) as well.

1 medium onion, chopped finely
2 large carrots, sliced thinly
1lb (450g) chicken breast, skin and fat removed and
    diced
1 can (10.4oz/295g) Weight Watchers from Heinz
    Chicken Noodle Soup
4oz (100g) frozen peas
1 tbsp chopped parsley
2 bay leaves
Salt and black pepper
1½lb (675g) boiling potatoes (peeled weight), cooked and
    mashed with a little skimmed milk
3 slices Weight Watchers from Heinz Reduced Fat
    Processed Cheese, chopped finely
Parsley to garnish

1.   Cook the onion and carrot in a little water until soft. Add the diced chicken and continue cooking until the meat turns white.
2.   Drain off the water, add the soup to the chicken, bring to the boil, cover and simmer gently for 10 minutes.
3.   Add the peas, parsley, bay leaves and seasoning to taste. Cover and simmer gently for 5 minutes. Discard the bay leaves.

4. Meanwhile, prepare the potatoes, then mix two thirds of the chopped cheese with the mashed potato, and season to taste.
5. Put the chicken mixture into a deep ovenproof dish, and fork or pipe the potato on top.
6. Sprinkle with the remaining chopped cheese.
7. Bake at 375°F, 190°C, gas mark 5 for 25–30 minutes. The potato should be browned on top. Garnish with parsley sprigs just before serving.

GAMMON STEAKS WITH PINEAPPLE AND MUSTARD SAUCE

Serves: 4
Calories per serving: 225

This is scrumptious served with a couple of large grilled tomatoes, green beans and a green salad . . . for hardly any extra calories!

4 3oz (75g) lean gammon steaks, fat trimmed off
4 pineapple rings, canned in juice, and drained
1 small carton (5oz/150g) natural, low-fat yogurt
½ tsp made-up English mustard
½ tsp yeast extract
Salt and black pepper
2 tbsp chopped parsley
Parsley sprigs to garnish

1. Place the gammon steaks in a shallow ovenproof dish, and top each one with a pineapple ring.
2. Mix together the remaining ingredients except the parsley garnish, and pour over the ham and pineapple.
3. Cook in a moderate oven (325°F, 170°C, gas mark 3) for 30 minutes. Garnish with parsley sprigs.

LOW CALORIE FISH AND CHIPS

Serves: 4
Calories per serving: 360

You can prepare this meal so quickly that it's hardly worth going to the chippie! What's more, you save about 600 calories!

1½lb (675g) cod or plaice fillets
1 small carton (5oz/150g) natural, low-fat yogurt
4oz (100g) wholemeal breadcrumbs
Salt and black pepper
12oz (350g) oven chips
1 lemon, cut into 4 wedges

1.   Dip the non-skin side of each fillet into the yogurt, then press in seasoned breadcrumbs, coating well.
2.   Lay the fish skinside down on a rack on a flat baking tray and bake in a very hot oven (475°F, 240°C, gas mark 9) for about 20 minutes, or until crisp and golden.
3.   Meanwhile, cook the chips according to the instructions on the packet.
4.   Serve the fish and chips with lemon wedges.

CHAPTER FOURTEEN

SPECIAL OCCASION MENUS

Fancy eating gourmet meals with friends and sticking to your diet? You can do it, if *you* do the entertaining! It's easy to take control of your own calorie intake if you are the one who's in the kitchen.

But no one wants to slave over a hot stove all night, so these recipes are simple, as well as impressive and low in calories. Should you tell your guests they are 'slimming' menus? That's up to you, but my advice is to wait until the end of the meal when their tummies are full. They'll never believe you!

Here are the menus in this chapter:

DINNER PARTY FOR SIX

Menu:

Salmon Pâté with toast triangles
Chicken Marsala with fluffy rice and crisp green salad
Ginger fruit salad

Calories per serving:

Salmon Pâté: *105 (175* with two wholemeal toast triangles)
Chicken Marsala: *365 (465* with 2 heaped tablespoons of plain, boiled rice)
Ginger Fruit Salad: *85*

This is a delicious, filling dinner. For your guests, you can add butter to go with the pâté, a cheese course, and thin biscuits to nibble with the fruit salad. The starter and dessert can be made in advance and kept in the fridge until needed.

SALMON PÂTÉ

1 small can (3.7oz/105g) red salmon, drained
4oz (100g) low-fat Cheddar cheese, grated finely
2 tsp lemon juice
2 tsp Worcestershire sauce
2 tbsp reduced-calorie mayonnaise
Grated rind of ¼ lemon
1 tbsp finely chopped parsley
1 tbsp chopped nuts
Cucumber and lemon slices to garnish

1.   Beat all the ingredients together.
2.   Chill and serve in small ramekin dishes or on a large platter garnished with cucumber and lemon slices, plus triangles of toast.

CHICKEN MARSALA

6 chicken breasts (8oz/225g each)
Seasoned flour
1 tbsp corn oil
6oz (175g) button mushrooms, sliced
2 tsp flour
5fl oz (150ml) dry white wine
3 tbsp Marsala wine
1 small carton (3½oz/100g) low-fat, natural fromage frais
Salt and black pepper
4oz (100g) Edam cheese, cut into six slices
1oz (25g) flaked almonds, toasted, to garnish
Chopped fresh parsley to garnish

1.   Remove the skin and any bones from the chicken breasts and coat in the seasoned flour.
2.   Put the oil in a large, heavy-based, non-stick pan, and cook the breasts gently, turning occasionally, for about 15–20 minutes until golden brown and cooked through.
3.   Remove from the pan, place in an ovenproof serving dish and keep warm in a low oven.
4.   Sauté the mushrooms in the pan, and add to the chicken. Sprinkle the flour in the pan, cook for 1 minute, blending with the bits left in the pan. Gradually add the white wine and Marsala. Bring to the boil, stirring constantly.
5.   Add the fromage frais and reheat gently. Do not boil. Season to taste.
6.   Poor the sauce over the chicken and place the slices of Edam on top. Brown under a hot grill. Sprinkle with toasted almonds and chopped parsley and serve.

GINGER FRUIT SALAD

1 large Ogen melon
8oz (225g) grapes
8oz (225g) fresh or frozen raspberries
Juice of 1 orange
1 tbs sherry
Pinch of ground ginger
1 small carton (5oz/150g) natural, low-fat yogurt to
   decorate
6 pieces preserved ginger to decorate

1. Cut the melon in half and remove the seeds. Cut the flesh into balls with a small teaspoon or use a melon baller if you have one.
2. Cut the grapes in half and remove the pips.
3. Place all the fruit in a bowl.
4. Mix together the orange juice, sherry and ground ginger.
5. Pour over the fruit, place in the fridge and leave to soak for several hours.
6. Spoon into small glass dishes and top each with a spoonful of yogurt and a piece of preserved ginger.

LOVERS' DINNER

Menu:
      Cucumber and Strawberry Salad
      Pork Chops with Rosemary and Orange Sauce
      Fresh Pineapple and Rum Surprise
Calories per serving:
      Cucumber and Strawberry Salad: *25*
      Pork Chops with Rosemary and Orange Sauce: *290*
      Pineapple and Rum Surprise: *120*

*If you want to get your partner in the mood for love, give him
– or her – this delicious supper. It's light, tasty, low in
calories and packed with vitamins and minerals so you'll
both feel frisky when you finish the meal! What's more, you
can have a couple of glasses of bubbly with your supper and
still stick to your diet!*

CUCUMBER AND STRAWBERRY SALAD

½ small cucumber, peeled and sliced very thinly
6 strawberries, sliced
1 tbsp dry white wine
Dash of white wine vinegar
Salt and black pepper
Mint sprigs to garnish

1.   Arrange the cucumber slices in a heart shape on a
large plate.
2.   Fill in the centre with the slices of strawberry.
3.   Mix together the wine, vinegar and salt and black
pepper to taste. Spoon over the salad, cover and chill.
Serve garnished with sprigs of mint.

PORK CHOPS WITH ROSEMARY AND ORANGE SAUCE

2 oranges
2 lean pork chops (about 8oz/225g), trimmed of fat
1 tsp dried rosemary
Salt and black pepper

1.   Peel and slice 1 orange and squeeze the juice from the other orange.
2.   Grill the chops until brown on both sides under a medium heat on a rack so any fat drips through and can be discarded. Keep the chops warm on a serving dish.
3.   Meanwhile, heat the orange juice in a small pan with the rosemary. Add the orange slices, and heat through.
4.   Pour the sauce over the chops and serve at once, with a crisp green salad and plenty of 'free' vegetables (*see* page 35).

FRESH PINEAPPLE AND RUM SURPRISE

1 small pineapple
1 dsp Hermesetas Sprinkle Sweet
2 tbsp dark rum
1 kiwi fruit, sliced

1.   Cut the pineapple into quarters, lengthwise, removing the core, but reserving the leaves.
2.   Arrange the quarters attractively on a serving plate.
3.   Mix the Sprinkle Sweet and rum together and pour over the pineapple.
4.   Decorate with sliced kiwi fruit and serve.

CHRISTMAS DINNER FOR EIGHT

Menu:

Prawn and Grapefruit Cocktail with Seafood Sauce

Roast Turkey with Prune and Apple Stuffing, Sprouts, Green Beans, Bread Sauce, Roast Potatoes and Carrots

Oranges in Grand Marnier

Calories per serving:

Prawn and Grapefruit Cocktail with Seafood Sauce: *150*

Roast Turkey with Prune and Apple Stuffing (average serving): *360*

Oranges in Grand Marnier: *120*

There is no doubt that Christmas lunch is the biggest blowout of the year. It is quite possible to consume 3000 calories at one meal, if you have lashings of stuffing, roast potatoes, pud, cream, chocs, wine and liqueurs. However, if you stick to this basic menu, with a couple of glasses of dry wine, and a small chunk of roast potato and thin gravy you'll stay within 1000 calories. Remember to pile 'free' vegetables like sprouts and green beans on your plate (page 35). My recipe for Turkey Mayonnaise on page 221 is the best one I know for 'recycling' leftover turkey. I usually make a big dish of it for our Boxing Day buffet supper. If you add a crisp salad, and a small baked potato, with fruit to follow, you'll still have change from 450 calories.

PRAWN AND GRAPEFRUIT COCKTAIL WITH SEAFOOD SAUCE

4 pink grapefruit
1lb (450g) peeled prawns
Salad leaves to line the bowls
Sprigs of mint to garnish
Sauce
4 tbsp reduced-calorie mayonnaise
4 tbsp natural, low-fat yogurt
8 tsp tomato ketchup
2–3 drops hot pepper sauce

1.   Peel the grapefruit and remove the pith. Cut between the membranes to remove the segments, and cut each one in half.
2.   Mix the prawns and grapefruit segments together.
3.   Line 8 small bowls with salad leaves and divide the prawn and grapefruit mixture between them.
4.   Mix together the sauce ingredients, adding the hot pepper sauce last – don't add too much. Chill until needed.
5.   Spoon the seafood sauce on top of the prawn and grapefruit cocktail and garnish with sprigs of fresh mint.

ROAST TURKEY WITH PRUNE AND APPLE STUFFING

1 6lb (2.7kg) turkey, fresh or thoroughly defrosted
12oz (350g) fresh breadcrumbs
24 prunes, soaked overnight in water, stoned and
    chopped
4 large apples, cored and chopped
Grated rind and juice of 2 lemons
2 small eggs (size 4), beaten
A little skimmed milk
Salt and black pepper

1.   Mix the breadcrumbs, prunes, pieces of apple and
lemon rind. Add the beaten egg and lemon juice to bind the
mixture. If necessary add a little milk, depending on how
dry you like your stuffing! Season to taste.
2.   Stuff the turkey neck with the mixture, place in a
roasting tin with a little water in the bottom and roast in a
hot oven (400°F, 200°C, gas mark 6) for about 3 hours,
basting frequently.
3.   Serve with green vegetables and carrots (no butter on
top, please!), and large chunks of potato roasted the
Fatfield way (brush parboiled potatoes with vegetable oil,
and brown under the grill).

ORANGES IN GRAND MARNIER

8 oranges
6fl oz (175ml) water
4oz (100g) runny honey
3 tbsp lemon juice
4fl oz (100ml) Grand Marnier

1.   Using a vegetable peeler, peel thin strips of rind from 3 of the oranges.
2.   Peel all the oranges, and remove the white pith. Cut the oranges into round slices and arrange, overlapping, on a serving dish.
3.   In a small saucepan, combine the water and honey. Bring to the boil, add the orange rind and lemon juice. Simmer for 5 minutes. Remove from the heat, and stir in the Grand Marnier.
4.   Pour over the oranges and chill until required.

BOXING DAY TURKEY MAYONNAISE

Serves: 6
Calories per serving: 220

The hint of curry in the sauce satisfies the lust of Christmas guests who are already planning to sneak off to the local Indian restaurant, rather than face yet more cold meat!

1 small onion, chopped
1 clove garlic
4fl oz (100ml) water
1 tbsp tomato purée
½ tsp curry powder
2 tbsp lemon juice
2 tbsp low-sugar apricot jam
4 tbsp reduced-calorie mayonnaise
4 tbsp natural, low-fat yogurt
1lb (450g) cooked, diced turkey
8oz (225g) grapes, green and black
1½oz (40g) flaked almonds
Watercress to garnish

1.   Simmer the onion and garlic in the water with the tomato purée, curry powder and 1 tablespoon of lemon juice for 8 minutes.
2.   Place in a blender with the jam, and blend until smooth. Allow to cool.
3.   In a large bowl, mix the mayonnaise, yogurt and onion mixture. Stir in the diced turkey and chill.
4.   Just before serving, toss the grapes in the remaining tablespoon of lemon juice and stir into the turkey mayonnaise.
5.   Brown the flaked almonds under the grill.
6.   Pile the turkey mixture onto a serving dish, and garnish with the almonds and watercress.

BUFFET PARTY FOR TEN

Menu:
Chicken Tandoori with Yogurt and Cucumber
Cold Ratatouille
Ham and Beansprout Salad
Green Salad with Lemon Vinaigrette Dressing
Fish Pie with Crunchy Topping
Red Fruit Salad
Cherry Yogurt Icecream

Calories per serving:
Chicken Tandoori with Yogurt and Cucumber: *200*
Cold Ratatouille: *35*
Ham and Beansprout Salad: *110*
Green Salad with Lemon Vinaigrette Dressing: *20*
Fish Pie with Crunchy Topping: *235*
Red Fruit Salad: *60*
Cherry Yogurt Icecream: *115*

The easiest, and cheapest way to cater for a crowd is to serve up a buffet supper. Slimmers usually find that the main pitfalls they face are nibbles like nuts, canapés, and the cheese board.

But with this menu, anyone watching their weight can feel confident that they can eat well and stick to their diet. In fact, you could choose a huge plateful from these goodies for less than 500 calories.

Don't forget to get plenty of soda and sparkling mineral water so your guests can have 'spritzers' instead of straight white wine. It's easy to double, or treble quantities if you are planning a bigger bash.

CHICKEN TANDOORI WITH YOGURT AND CUCUMBER

2 small pieces fresh root ginger, peeled and chopped
4 cloves garlic, peeled and chopped
4 black peppercorns
2 tsp chilli powder
2 tsp ground coriander
1 tsp ground cumin
½ tsp salt
Finely grated rind and juice of 1 lemon
1–2 drops red food colouring
10 chicken breasts, about 6oz (175g) each, skinned
4 small cartons (5oz/150g) natural, low-fat yogurt
Lettuce and tomatoes to garnish
1 cucumber, sliced thinly

1. Pound the ginger, garlic and peppercorns in a pestle and mortar or use the back of a tablespoon in a small saucepan. Mix with the chilli powder, ground coriander and cumin, salt, lemon rind and juice and red colouring.
2. Score the chicken 3 times across each breast with a sharp knife, then rub with the tandoori mixture, pressing well into the flesh.
3. Coat each chicken breast with 1 tablespoon yogurt, and chill for 24 hours.
4. Cook under a medium grill, turning once, until the chicken is cooked through and the outside is dark red-brown.
5. Arrange the lettuce and tomato garnish on a large platter and place the chicken on top.
6. Serve the remaining yogurt separately, with cucumber slices floating on top.

COLD RATATOUILLE

2 large aubergines, sliced
Salt
2 large onions, sliced finely
2 large cans (14oz/397g) tomatoes
2 cloves garlic, peeled and crushed
2 large green or red peppers, cored, deseeded and sliced
    finely
1½lb (675g) courgettes, sliced
1 tsp dried mixed herbs
1 tsp tomato purée
Salt and black pepper

1.   Sprinkle the aubergine slices with salt. Leave to stand for 20 minutes, then rinse with cold water and pat dry with kitchen paper.
2.   Place the onion and aubergine slices in a large, heavy-based, non-stick pan and pour over the tomatoes. Add the garlic and simmer gently for 5 minutes.
3.   Add the peppers and courgettes, stir, cover and simmer for 15 minutes or until the vegetables are cooked but not mushy. Add a little water if necessary.
4.   Stir in the herbs and tomato purée, and simmer for a further 5 minutes.
5.   Remove from the heat, season to taste and pour into a serving dish.
6.   Chill before serving.

HAM AND BEANSPROUT SALAD

8oz (225g) lean ham, cut into strips
1 large cucumber, peeled and cut into 1in (2.5cm) strips
1 small red and 1 small green pepper, cored, deseeded
    and diced finely
1lb (450g) beansprouts, canned or fresh
3 large oranges, peeled, pith removed and cut into
    segments
1 large lettuce, shredded
1 tbsp chopped chives
Dressing
1oz (25g) Danish Blue cheese, crumbled
3oz (75g) Shape Low Fat Soft Cheese
3 tbsp natural, low-fat yogurt

1.   In a large bowl, mix together the ham, cucumber,
peppers, beansprouts and orange segments.
2.   Arrange the shredded lettuce in a serving dish, and
pile the salad in the centre.
3.   Make the dressing by mixing the Danish Blue cheese
with the Soft Cheese and yogurt.
4.   Pour the dressing over the salad and garnish with
chopped chives.

GREEN SALAD WITH LEMON VINAIGRETTE DRESSING

1 large lettuce
4oz (100g) spinach, washed and thick stalks removed
1 curly endive
1 cucumber, sliced thinly
12 spring onions, trimmed and chopped finely
4 sticks celery, chopped finely
1 tbsp each chopped tarragon, thyme and parsley to
  garnish
Dressing
4 tbsp wine vinegar
4 tbsp lemon juice
1 tsp Dijon mustard
1 clove garlic, peeled and crushed (optional)
Salt and black pepper

1.   Line a salad bowl with lettuce leaves.
2.   Shred the remaining lettuce with the spinach and endive, and pile into the bowl.
3.   Arrange the cucumber slices on top and scatter over the chopped spring onions and celery.
4.   Mix together the dressing ingredients.
5.   Scatter the chopped herbs on top of the salad, and toss with the dressing just before serving.

FISH PIE WITH CRUNCHY TOPPING

1lb (450g) carrots, sliced
1lb (450g) leeks, sliced
2 celery hearts, sliced
2lb (900g) boiling potatoes (peeled weight), sliced
1 small carton (5oz/150g), natural, low-fat yogurt
Salt and black pepper
3lb (1.3kg) white fish fillet (e.g. cod, coley)
2 cans (10.4oz/295g) reduced-calorie celery or
    mushroom soup
A little skimmed milk
2lb (900g) tomatoes, sliced
6 tsp Bran Flakes
Parsley sprigs to garnish

1.   Cook the carrots, leeks and celery hearts in boiling water until tender but still crunchy. Drain.
2.   Cook the potatoes until tender, drain and mash with the yogurt. Season to taste.
3.   Simmer the fish in water for 10 minutes. Strain, remove any skin and bones and flake the fish into large chunks.
4.   Pour the soup into a bowl, and blend gently with the fish, carrots, leeks and celery hearts, adding a little skimmed milk if necessary. Adjust the seasoning.
5.   Pile the fish and vegetable mixture into a 3 pint (1.8 litre) pie dish, cover with the tomatoes and spread the mashed potato on top.
6.   Bake in a hot oven (400°F, 200°C, gas mark 6) for 30 minutes, sprinkle on the Bran Flakes and return to the oven for 5 minutes.
7.   Serve garnished with parsley sprigs.

RED FRUIT SALAD

You can, of course, use other red fruits according to what is in season.

4 crisp red apples
2 tbsp lemon juice
8oz (225g) blackberries
8oz (225g) raspberries
8oz (225g) strawberries
8oz (225g) red cherries, stoned
4 large red plums, stoned and chopped
2 tbsp dry sherry
2 tbsp unsweetened apple juice
2 tsp Hermesetas Sprinkle Sweet
Mint leaves to garnish

1.   Core and slice the apples, and cover with lemon juice to prevent discolouring.
2.   Combine all the fruit in a bowl.
3.   Mix together the sherry, apple juice and Sprinkle Sweet.
4.   Pour over the fruit, chill, and serve garnished with mint.

CHERRY YOGURT ICECREAM

1 large can (15oz/425g) black cherries, canned in syrup
½pt (275ml) Shape Double
2 small cartons (4½oz/125g) low-calorie Black Cherry
   Yogurt
2 egg whites

1.   Drain the cherries, reserving the syrup, and remove the stones.
2.   Purée the cherries and syrup.
3.   Whip the Double until it holds its shape, and beat in the yogurt and cherry purée.
4.   Whisk the egg whites until stiff, and then fold into the cherry cream.
5.   Place in a large freezerproof container.
6.   Freeze for about 3 hours, then remove and beat before returning to the freezer.
7.   Remove from the freezer about 30 minutes before serving and place in the fridge to soften slightly.

CURRY SUPPER FOR FOUR

Menu:
  Cucumber Raita
  Quick Keema

Calories per serving:
  Cucumber Raita: *45*
  Quick Keema: *About 265*

Instead of sending out for a takeaway, save cash (and calories) with a home-cooked curry supper. This simple menu, served with salad and some crisp white wine or lager is ideal for a Friday or Saturday night, when you want to entertain friends without working too hard!

CUCUMBER RAITA

4oz (100g) cucumber, sliced thinly
Salt
2 small cartons (5oz/150g) natural, low-fat yogurt
2oz (50g) spring onions, sliced thinly
1 green chilli, deseeded and chopped finely
Coriander leaves to garnish

1.   Place the cucumber slices in a colander, sprinkle with salt and leave to drain for 30 minutes. Dry thoroughly.
2.   Mix the yogurt with salt to taste and fold in the cucumber, spring onions and chilli.
3.   Place in a serving dish, garnish with coriander leaves and chill until required.

QUICK KEEMA

The Quick Keema is a very easy curry dish which can be prepared in advance and frozen. In fact, many cooks (and I'm one of them) believe that freezing actually improves the flavour of curry. Fatfield slimmer Linda Philpott sometimes adds quartered potatoes and shelled peas to this dish to make it even more substantial.

1lb (450g) lean minced beef
1 medium onion, sliced finely
1 green chilli, deseeded and sliced finely
2 cloves garlic, crushed
Pinch of turmeric
1 tsp each chilli, coriander and cumin powder
1 large can (14oz/397g) chopped tomatoes
4oz (100g) frozen peas
1 tbsp cornflour
1 small carton (5oz/150g) natural, low-fat yogurt

1.   'Dry fry' the minced beef in a large, heavy-based, non-stick saucepan, stirring until the meat changes colour. Drain off all the fat.
2.   Add the onion, chilli, garlic, spices and tomatoes. Cover and cook gently for about 20 minutes.
3.   Add the peas and cook for a further 5 minutes.
4.   Mix the cornflour with a little cold water to make a smooth paste. Stir into the saucepan with the yogurt. Cook, stirring all the time, for 2 minutes, then serve.

KIDS' BUFFET PARTY FOR EIGHT

Menu:
> Wholemeal Pizza Rolls
> Cottage Cheese and Banana Muffins
> Low-Fat Crisps and Vegetable Medley with Three
> Dips
> Apricot Chiffon Pie

Calories per serving:
> Wholemeal Pizza Rolls: *245*
> Cottage Cheese and Banana Muffins: *190*
> Low-Fat Crisps and Vegetable Medley with Three
> Dips: *70*
> Apricot Chiffon Pie: *190*

Nowadays, children have sophisticated tastes. They are more likely to go for savoury titbits like crisps and pizza than traditional kiddy favourites like jelly and icecream.

This menu is tasty and cuts back on calories – so mums and dads can tuck in too. More important, it also cuts down fat and provides plenty of fibre. Add fruit 'kebabs' (chunks of fresh or canned fruit such as grapes or pineapple cubes, stuck on skewers), and homemade lemonade or a non-alcoholic punch to drink.

WHOLEMEAL PIZZA ROLLS

8 2oz (50g) soft wholemeal rolls
1 clove garlic
Pinch of salt
2 tsp low-fat spread
4 tbsp tomato purée
16 slices Weight Watchers from Heinz Reduced Fat
    Processed Cheese
1 dsp dried oregano or thyme
8 drained, canned anchovy fillets, sliced
8 stuffed olives, sliced

1. Cut the rolls in half.
2. Crush the garlic with the salt and work into the low-fat spread.
3. Spread both halves of the rolls with the spread and toast under the grill until lightly browned.
4. Spread each half with tomato purée and top each half with 1 cheese slice. Sprinkle lightly with oregano or thyme. Garnish with slices of anchovy and stuffed olives.
5. Just before serving, replace the rolls under the grill until the cheese bubbles.

COTTAGE CHEESE AND BANANA MUFFINS

8 wholemeal muffins
1oz (25g) low-fat spread
A little Marmite
2 bananas
2 tbsp lemon juice
8oz (225g) cottage cheese
1 punnet cress

1. Split the muffins and toast under the grill.
2. Spread with low-fat spread and Marmite.
3. Slice the bananas, and toss in lemon juice to prevent discolouring.
4. Top each muffin half with a spoonful of cottage cheese, a sprinkling of cress and a few banana slices.
5. Replace the tops, and garnish with the rest of the cress.

LOW FAT CRISPS AND VEGETABLE MEDLEY WITH THREE DIPS

2 packets Low-Fat Crisps
Selection of washed and prepared vegetables, cut into
  bite-size pieces – e.g. cucumber, cauliflower, red and
  green peppers, carrot and celery sticks
1 carton (5oz/150g) Shape Onion and Chives Soft Cheese
1 small carton (5oz/150g) natural, low-fat yogurt
2 spring onions, chopped finely
1 tsp lemon juice
1 tsp each ginger and curry powder
½ tsp paprika
A few drops of Tabasco Sauce
6 tbsp Heidelberg Calorie Reduced Thousand Island
  Dressing
Lemon slices and parsley to garnish

1.   Arrange the crisps and vegetables attractively on
small plates.
2.   To make the cheese and onion dip, mix Shape Onion
and Chives Soft Cheese with 1 tablespoon yogurt, 2 spring
onions and the lemon juice.
3.   To make the curry dip, mix the remaining yogurt with
the curry powder, ginger and paprika, and add Tabasco to
taste.
4.   For the third dip, pour Heidelberg dressing into a
small bowl.
5.   Place the cheese and curry dips in small bowls and
garnish.

APRICOT CHIFFON PIE

4oz (100g) digestive biscuits
2oz (50g) butter
1 large can (15oz/425g) apricots, canned in natural juice
2 tsp powdered gelatine
2 tbsp Hermesetas Sprinkle Sweet
4fl oz (100ml) evaporated milk
1oz (25g) plain or milk chocolate to decorate

1. Crush the biscuits. Melt the butter and mix with the biscuit crumbs.
2. Press into an 8in (20cm) flan case and chill until needed.
3. Drain the apricots and reserve the juice. Place 4 tablespoons of the juice in a small basin and sprinkle the gelatine on the juice. Leave to soak for 5 minutes until spongy. Stand the basin in a pan containing a little simmering water and leave until the gelatine has dissolved.
4. Purée the apricots with another 4 tablespoons of juice and the Sprinkle Sweet.
5. Add the dissolved gelatine and stir well.
6. Whisk the evaporated milk until foamy.
7. Add the purée and continue to whisk for another minute.
8. Pour into the flan case, chill, and decorate with grated chocolate when set.

CHAPTER FIFTEEN

LOW-CALORIE CONTINENTAL CLASSICS

One of the surprising things about foreign travel is watching the locals tucking into calorie-laden meals without putting on weight. Chic French women seem to manage to stay trim on a diet of *pommes frites* and runny cheese, gorgeous Italians can wolf down pasta at every meal without putting on an ounce, and even Spanish waiters stay slinky-hipped on platefuls of paella!

The truth is that most Europeans don't eat their most fattening national dishes every day – and when they do indulge in a high-calorie main course, they invariably follow it with fresh fruit or a simple sorbet.

What's more, even classic Continental cooks are now looking for ways of preparing dishes with fewer fatty ingredients. They're swapping double cream for yogurt or *crème fraîche*, cutting back on butter, and simplifying the rich sauces that used to double or treble the fattening power of fish and meat.

Here's a selection of some of the most popular European dishes, specially for slimmers. They're simple to cook, delicious, and will recapture the magic of those holidays abroad.

FRANCE

COQ-AU-VIN

Serves: 4
Calories per serving: 280

This is a cheapish dinner party dish that looks and tastes really special. Of course, if you are feeling flush, you can upgrade the wine you use – it will make a difference to the price, but won't affect the calories. Serve the coq-au-vin with plain boiled rice and a salad.

4 medium (9oz/250g) chicken leg portions
½ pt (275ml) chicken stock
8oz (225g) button onions, peeled or large onions, peeled and sliced
8oz (225g) button mushrooms
Chopped parsley to garnish
Marinade
2 cloves garlic, crushed (optional)
1 bay leaf
½pt (275ml) red wine
Salt and black pepper

1. Skin the chicken and place in a shallow dish.
2. Mix the marinade ingredients, season to taste, and pour over the chicken. Cover and marinade in the fridge for 3 hours.
3. Remove the chicken from the marinade. Reserve the marinade.
4. Place the chicken in an ovenproof casserole dish, and brown under a hot grill, turning once.
5. Pour the chicken stock over the chicken, add the onions, cover and cook in a moderate oven (350°F, 180°C,

gas mark 4) for about 1½ hours. Add the mushrooms, and cook for a further 20 minutes.

6.   Discard the bay leaf and pour the marinade into a small saucepan. Boil for about 5 minutes to reduce and thicken slightly, then pour over the casserole. Garnish with chopped parsley before serving.

SALAD NIÇOISE

Serves: 4
Calories per serving: 120

4 anchovy fillets
1 clove garlic, cut in half
1lb (450g) new potatoes
1 tbsp oil-free, low-calorie vinaigrette
1 tsp chopped parsley
Salt and black pepper
12 black olives
4 medium, firm tomatoes, quartered
1 small onion, sliced thinly

1.   Wash the anchovy fillets under running water and cut each one into three.
2.   Rub a salad bowl with the cut garlic clove.
3.   Boil and peel the potatoes, slice while still warm and place in the salad bowl. Mix the vinaigrette, parsley and seasoning and pour over the warm potatoes. Toss lightly.
4.   When cool, stir in the olives, anchovy pieces, tomatoes and sliced onion.

MOULES MARINIÈRES

Serves: 2
Calories per serving: 290

Mussels are so easy to prepare and low in calories (about 25 per 1oz/25g shelled weight) that it's surprising that slimmers don't eat them more often. The problem is usually availability, and the fact that it's necessary to eat them the very same day you buy them.

Nowadays, more supermarkets have fresh fish counters with mussels on display. Try them for a treat after a late-night shopping spree. They are incredibly quick to cook, and taste wonderful with bread and a couple of glasses of the cooking wine!

4 pints (2.3 litres) fresh mussels on the shell
2 shallots or 1 medium onion, chopped
4 stalks parsley
1 sprig thyme
Black pepper
¼pt (150ml) dry white wine
¼pt (150ml) water
Chopped parsley to garnish

1.   Scrape and clean the mussels in several changes of cold water, discarding any that are not tightly shut.
2.   Put the cleaned mussels into a wide pan with the shallots, herbs, freshly ground pepper, wine and water. Cover the pan and cook over a high heat for 5–6 minutes, shaking the pan occasionally. Discard any mussels that do not open.
3.   As soon as the mussels open, place them on warm plates.
4.   Strain the liquid over the mussels and sprinkle with chopped parsley.

ITALY

FETTUCCINE WITH SMOKED SALMON

Serves: 6 as a starter, 4 as a main course
Calories: 330 or 490

This recipe is often served as a starter in Italian restaurants, smothered in cream! However, it is just as good with natural yogurt and unsweetened fromage frais instead of the cream, and is quite cheap to make if you use smoked salmon 'ends' which you can buy in most supermarkets.

10oz (275g) smoked salmon slices or 'ends'
3 tbsp natural, low-fat yogurt
3 tbsp unsweetened fromage frais, 8 per cent fat
12oz (350g) fettuccine
Black pepper

1.   Cut the salmon into 1in (2.5cm) strips. Mix the yogurt with the fromage frais.
2.   Place the salmon in a bowl, and pour over the yogurt mixture. Leave to stand for about 2 hours.
3.   Cook the pasta in plenty of boiling, salted water until 'al dente' – cooked but still firm with a touch of bite to it.
4.   Heat the salmon mixture in a heavy saucepan over very low heat. Do not allow it to boil.
5.   Pour over the pasta and stir. Season with freshly ground black pepper and serve at once.

SPAGHETTI BOLOGNESE

Serves 4
Calories per serving: 390

It's convenient to use a ready-made sauce for Bolognese, but this can bump up calories alarmingly, once you include the minced beef and the cheese on top.

For instance, a popular commercial red wine and herb sauce 'costs' 350 calories per four servings, compared with under 50 for the homemade kind.

Use the Quick Tomato Sauce recipe on page 258 if you like, or try this version which is closer to the traditional sauce and tastes wonderful. Instead of spaghetti you can also use tagliatelle which is traditionally served in Bologna in north-ern Italy where this dish originated.

Bolognese Sauce
2oz (50g) lean, unsmoked bacon, chopped finely
1 small onion, chopped finely
8oz (225g) lean minced beef
1 large can (14oz/397g) chopped tomatoes
2oz (50g) carrot, chopped finely
1 stick celery, chopped finely
6 tbsp dry white wine
¼pt (150ml) beef stock or water
Salt and black pepper
Pinch of nutmeg

Pasta
8oz (225g) spaghetti or tagliatelle
1 tbsp grated Parmesan cheese

1.   Dry fry the bacon over a low heat in a heavy based, non-stick pan until it starts to colour.
2.   Add the onion and beef, stirring well to prevent stick-

ing. Continue cooking for a few minutes, then drain off any fat, and transfer the mixture to a large saucepan.
3.   Add the chopped tomatoes, carrot and celery and cook gently for 15 minutes.
4.   Add the wine, stock or water, salt, freshly ground black pepper and a pinch of nutmeg. Stir, cover the saucepan and simmer gently for 30 minutes, stirring occasionally.
5.   Remove from the heat, check the seasoning and serve.
6.   Meanwhile, boil the spaghetti or tagliatelle in plenty of lightly salted water until cooked but 'al dente' or firm with a touch of bite to it. Drain and serve, topped with the sauce and grated Parmesan cheese.

STEAK PIZZAIOLA

Serves: 2
Calories per serving: 350

This recipe makes rump steak taste very special, and is a great choice for a dinner party. Add noodles for your guests, plus a selection of green vegetables from your 'free' list (see page 35).

2 thin rump steaks, about 5oz (150g) each
Salt and black pepper
½ recipe Quick Tomato Sauce (page 258), heated through

1.   Season the steaks with salt and freshly ground black pepper, and place on a rack. Grill on each side under a high heat until cooked.
2.   Transfer to an ovenproof dish, pour the sauce over, and serve.

SPAIN

GAZPACHO

Serves: 4
Calories per serving: 65

This is a perfect summer soup, and so low in calories that you can drink as much as you like. If you prefer a smoother soup put the canned tomatoes in the blender and add the chilled tomato juice afterwards.

1 large cucumber
1 medium green pepper, cored and deseeded
1 medium red pepper, cored and deseeded
3 cloves garlic, chopped
2 tbsp wine vinegar
1½ pts (850ml) tomato juice, chilled
1 small can (8oz/227g) chopped tomatoes, chilled
Juice of ½ a lemon
Salt and black pepper

1.   Cut half the cucumber and peppers into tiny cubes and arrange on a serving dish, as a garnish.
2.   Roughly chop the remaining cucumber and peppers.
3.   Put in a blender with the garlic and wine vinegar. Liquidize until smooth. Stir into the chilled tomato juice.
4.   Finally stir in the chilled chopped tomatoes and lemon juice and season to taste.
5.   Serve in a large bowl, with ice cubes, handing the garnish separately.

SPANISH OMELETTE

Serves: 4
Calories per serving: 275

If you want to make good, low-calorie omelettes, you need a non-stick pan that really is non-stick – i.e. not an old one which has lost most of the non-stick coating. This family-sized version of a Spanish lunchtime favourite includes hardly any oil at all, but has all the taste of the original.

4oz (100g) potato, peeled and diced
2 medium onions, chopped
6 eggs
4oz (100g) lean ham, diced
2oz (50g) frozen peas
2oz (50g) sweetcorn
1 tsp corn oil
Salt and black pepper

1.   Place the diced potato and onion in a saucepan in a little water. Cook gently for about 15 minutes, until the onion is soft and the potatoes are cooked but still firm. Drain.
2.   Break the eggs into a bowl, beat with a fork just enough to blend the yolks and whites thoroughly. Add the potatoes and onion, ham, frozen peas and sweetcorn. Season lightly.
3.   Heat the oil in a large, heavy-based, non-stick pan, pour in the egg mixture and cook until the base is set, about 5 minutes, shaking the pan occasionally to prevent sticking.
4.   Finish cooking the top of the omelette under a high grill, until the top is brown. Serve cut into wedges.

PAELLA VALENCIANA

Serves: 4
Calories per serving: 435

There are many versions of paella, some using both meat and seafood, others with just seafood or vegetables. You can experiment with this basic recipe, adding or subtracting different ingredients.

If you can't afford the prawns and mussels, it's almost as tasty with chunks of tuna (canned in brine) and chopped, grilled low-fat sausage instead.

The main rule to follow is that the liquid should be double the volume of the rice, and allow about 2oz (50g) of rice for each person.

2 tsp vegetable oil
3 cloves garlic, chopped (optional)
1 medium onion, chopped
3 medium tomatoes, blanched, peeled and chopped or 1
    small can (8oz/227g) tomatoes
1 medium red pepper, cored, deseeded and sliced
4 chicken drumsticks
1 tsp paprika
8oz (225g) long grain white rice
½ tsp yellow food colouring or turmeric
1pt (575ml) chicken stock, seasoned
8oz (225g) frozen peas
8oz (225g) cooked, shelled shrimps or prawns
1pt (575ml) mussels, scrubbed and bearded
Lemon wedges and parsley sprigs to garnish

1.   Heat the oil in a large, deep, heavy-based, non-stick frying pan. Add the garlic, onion, tomatoes, red pepper and chicken pieces. Reduce the heat and add the paprika.

2.   Cook for 10 minutes, stirring occasionally to prevent sticking.

3.   Spread the rice evenly in the pan and stir briefly.

4.   Remove the pan from heat and add the food colouring or turmeric and the stock.

5.   Return to the heat, bring to the boil and add the peas. Cover with a lid or foil.

6.   Simmer gently over a low heat for 15 minutes, or until the rice has cooked and almost all of the stock has been absorbed. Add the shrimps or prawns. If necessary, add a little extra water to prevent the rice sticking while cooking.

7.   Put the mussels on top of the rice, cover and cook for about 5 minutes or until the mussels open. Discard any that remain shut.

8.   Serve the paella hot, garnished with lemon wedges and parsley sprigs.

PORTUGAL

CALDO VERDE

Serves: 4
Calories per serving: 120

This soup is served as a starter in many Portuguese homes. It is an unusual way of serving good old cabbage and spuds, and is very tasty and filling. Recommended for lunch, with a crusty roll and fruit to follow.

2 pts (1.3 litres) water
4 medium potatoes, peeled and sliced
½ small cabbage, with coarse veins and leaves removed, shredded finely
Salt and black pepper
4 tbsp natural, low-fat yogurt
Paprika and a little chopped parsley to garnish

1.   Bring the water to the boil in a large saucepan, add the potatoes and salt to taste. Cover, reduce the heat and cook the potatoes until tender.
2.   Remove the potatoes, mash, return them to the pan and stir to mix.
3.   Add the shredded cabbage, bring the mixture to the boil, and cook for 5 minutes. Season to taste.
4.   Pour into four warmed soup bowls, add a spoonful of yogurt to each one, and sprinkle with paprika and chopped parsley.

PORTUGUESE COD

Serves: 4
Calories per serving: 280

1½lb (675g) cod fillet
1 large can (14oz/397g) chopped tomatoes
1 glass dry white wine
1 large onion, chopped finely
4oz (100g) long grain white rice
1 clove garlic, crushed
Parsley sprigs and lemon slices to garnish

1.   Place the tomatoes and wine in a saucepan, add the chopped onion, rice and garlic. Cover and cook gently until the rice is tender, about 15 minutes.
2.   Meanwhile, cut the fish into 4 cutlets and poach in a little water until cooked through but still firm. Drain and keep warm.
3.   Place the fish in a warmed serving dish, surround with the tomato and rice mixture, and garnish with parsley and lemon slices.

GREECE

BAKED STUFFED AUBERGINES

Serves: 4
Calories per serving: 80

Aubergines absorb oil very quickly indeed, which is why this Greek speciality is usually taboo for slimmers. For example, a 1oz (25g) aubergine slice contains just 4 calories, but fried in oil or fat, this figure zooms up to 60! Our version cuts out the oil completely, and is still yummy hot or cold.

2 large aubergines
2 tsp salt
¼pt (150ml) chicken stock
1 medium onion, chopped
1 clove garlic, crushed
3 tomatoes, skinned and chopped
1 tbsp chopped chives
1 tbsp sweetcorn
Salt and black pepper
1oz (25g) wholemeal breadcrumbs
1oz (25g) Edam cheese, grated

1.   Cut the aubergines in half lengthwise, slash the flesh and sprinkle with salt. Place, flat side down, on a plate and leave to drain for 1 hour. Rinse thoroughly, and pat dry with kitchen paper, then remove and chop the flesh, leaving the skins whole.
2.   Put 2 tablespoons of the stock into a non-stick pan, cover and cook the onion and garlic gently until soft. Add the aubergine flesh, tomatoes, chives, sweetcorn and seasoning to taste. Cook until the vegetables are soft, then pile into the aubergine cases.

3.   Place the aubergines in a shallow ovenproof dish. Mix together the breadcrumbs and cheese and sprinkle over the aubergines.
4.   Add the remaining stock to the dish, and cover with foil.
5.   Bake in a moderate oven (375°F, 190°C, gas mark 5) for 30 minutes. Serve hot or cold.

HUMMUS

Serves: 6
Calories per serving: 120

This is a simple-to-make starter which is delicious with pitta bread or crispbreads. Usually, the recipe includes olive oil, but this version tastes just as good and saves around 300 calories!

2 large cans (14oz/397g) chick peas
2 cloves garlic, crushed
2 tbsp lemon juice
1 tbsp sesame seeds
Salt and black pepper
Paprika and lemon slices to garnish

1.   Drain the chick peas, reserving the liquid, and put into a food processor or blender with 4fl oz (100ml) of the liquid.
2.   Add the garlic, lemon juice and sesame seeds.
3.   Blend until smooth and season to taste with salt and freshly ground black pepper.
4.   Garnish with paprika and lemon slices.

CHAPTER SIXTEEN

MICRO MAGIC

Microwave ovens are great for slimmers. Food can be cooked fast, without added fat, and imaginative dishes prepared in less time than it takes to raid the biscuit tin. You can defrost low-calorie meals like soups and casseroles rapidly, saving time and money.

For people who live alone or are alone at home during the day, micros are absolutely slimsational. While it seems time-consuming and wasteful to use a conventional oven to cook something for one person, it is quick, easy and economical to use the microwave. 'Instant' meals like baked potatoes topped with baked beans or cottage cheese, fresh fish with vegetables, nourishing thick soups are all filling and low in calories when cooked the micro way. You also save on washing up, because many meals can be eaten from the same dishes they are cooked in.

There are, of course, certain rules that must be followed by micro fans. It is vital to check that the food is cooked properly, particularly if it has been defrosted before cooking. Soups and casseroles should be stirred halfway through. Reheat food rapidly and thoroughly. Don't keep reheating it, you'll destroy vitamins and minerals. A ready-prepared dish being reheated should register at least 65°C (150°F), after you remove it from the micro. After standing time (during which the food carries on cooking), the temperature should rise by a few degrees. If in doubt, use a micro thermometer to check.

Covering food helps retain moisture, speeds up cooking

and prevents splatters in the oven. Cling film is often used to retain moisture on vegetables and casseroles, but you can use kitchen paper or paper napkins to cover baked potatoes – paper is porous and lets the steam escape. Don't forget to prick items like potatoes and low-fat sausages to prevent explosions!

These recipes are very simple and quick. They have been tried out by busy slimmers using a 650-watt microwave oven with a turntable. If your cooker is a higher wattage, decrease the cooking time slightly, and if it is lower, increase it. If it doesn't have a turntable, turn the dish once or twice during cooking.

INSTANT BREAKFAST

Serves: 1
Calories per serving: 220

Who says slimmers have to leap out of bed al dawn to cook breakfast? In just 2 minutes you can serve up this substantial high-fibre meal. Just add a glass of unsweetened orange juice and you'll be set up for the day. What's more, your diet won't be sabotaged by an attack of the mid-morning munchies!

1 slice wholemeal toast
1 small can (5.29oz/150g) baked beans
3 small tomatoes, halved
1 tbsp sweetcorn

1. Place the toast on a plate and pour the baked beans on top.
2. Arrange the tomatoes and sweetcorn around the toast.
3. Cook on High for 2 minutes.

PEARS WITH GINGER AND CHEESE STUFFING

Serves: 2
Calories per serving: 120

The combination of these three flavours is unusual, and delicious. Serve this for dessert, or for breakfast when you fancy a treat!

2 ginger biscuits
2oz (50g) skimmed milk soft cheese
2 medium pears, peeled, halved and cored
2 tbsp apple juice

1. Crush the biscuits and mix with the cheese.
2. Place the pear halves in a serving dish, hollow side up. Fill with the ginger and cheese mixture. Pour the apple juice around the pears.
3. Cover with cling film, pierce and microwave on High for 1½–2 minutes.

HOT SPICED GRAPEFRUIT

Serves: 2
Calories per serving: 15

This makes a change from the usual cold grapefruit starters. Serve it for Sunday brunch (with Boston Baked Beans, page 184, to follow), or before a rich-tasting main course at a dinner party.

1 grapefruit
1 tbsp Less Sharp PLJ Lemon Juice
1 tsp ground nutmeg
1 tsp ground cinnamon
Orange slices to garnish

1. Halve the grapefruit, and loosen the segments with a grapefruit knife.
2. Sprinkle with the PLJ and spices.
3. Place in 2 individual dishes, and cook on High for 2 minutes. Serve hot, garnished with orange slices.

MICRO CHIPS

Serves: 4
Calories per serving: 115

Just for a change, try making your own chips. It's very quick indeed in a micro, and they are guaranteed to be lovely and fresh! Get your grill very hot for the final browning. If you want posher, sauté potatoes, simply cut them into slices instead of chips and garnish with chopped parsley.

1lb (450g) potatoes, peeled weight
1 tbsp vegetable oil
Salt to taste

1. Peel, rinse and dry the potatoes, and cut into ½in (1cm) chips.
2. Place in an ovenproof dish, cover with kitchen paper and cook on High for 4 minutes. Stir and cook for a further 3 minutes.
3. Drain, pat dry with kitchen paper and brush with oil. Sprinkle with salt.
4. Brown the chips under a hot, preheated grill, turning to ensure even browning.

ITALIAN CAULIFLOWER

Serves: 4
Calories per serving: 110

This recipe has a delicious sauce which we have pared down to the minimum calorie count possible without sacrificing the taste. Add some noodles (no butter – you don't need it), if you're serving this as a supper dish and it's good on its own for lunch. Two greedy slimmers could share this and still get away with a 220-calorie lunchtime total!

1 large cauliflower
4 tbsp water
1 medium onion, chopped finely
1 large can (14oz/397g) tomatoes
4 stuffed olives, sliced
Pinch of marjoram
1 clove garlic, crushed (optional)
1 can (10.4oz/295g) low-calorie Chicken Soup
3 tbsp natural, low-fat yogurt
2oz (50g) low-fat Cheddar cheese, grated

1.   Wash the cauliflower and remove the outer green leaves. Break into large florets.
2.   Place in a large dish with the water, cover with perforated cling film and cook for 10 minutes on High. Move the florets around halfway through cooking.
3.   Place the onion in a bowl with 3 tablespoons of juice from the tomatoes. Cover and cook on High for 3 minutes.
4.   Add the olives, tomatoes, marjoram and garlic. Cover and cook on High for 2 minutes, stirring after 1 minute.
5.   Stir and pour over the cauliflower.
6.   Combine the soup and yogurt, pour over the cauliflower, sprinkle with cheese and cook on High for 2 minutes.

TEN-MINUTE CHILLI

Serves: 4
Calories per serving: 290

This is a warming treat on cold winter nights. Serve it, piping hot, in individual bowls with crusty bread or plain boiled rice and a crisp salad.

1 onion, chopped finely
1 green pepper, cored, deseeded and diced
12oz (350g) lean, minced beef
1 large can (15oz/425g) red kidney beans
4 tbsp liquid from the can
4 tbsp tomato purée
1 tsp chilli powder
½ tsp ground cumin
Salt and black pepper
Chopped parsley and cucumber slices

1.   Put the onion and green pepper into a 2pt (1.2 litre) casserole, cover and cook on High for 4 minutes to soften.
2.   Add the beef, bean liquid, tomato purée and chilli powder or cumin to taste. Stir thoroughly, cover with cling film, perforate and cook on High for 5 minutes.
3.   Remove from the oven, remove the cling film and stir. Cover again and cook for a further 3 minutes.
4.   Add the beans and stir well. Cook on High for 2 minutes.
5.   Season to taste with salt and freshly ground black pepper and serve garnished with parsley and cucumber slices.

QUICK TOMATO SAUCE

Serves: 6
Calories per serving: 20

You can make this up in larger quantities and keep it in the freezer until needed. I use it as a base for scrumptious low-calorie toppings for pasta (adding prawns, cooked chopped chicken, etc.) or with lean minced beef (dry-fried and drained of fat). I also like to toss finely chopped vegetables (e.g. courgettes, green beans or cauliflower) into a saucepan full of the sauce, to make a delicious lunchtime soup. The garlic is optional!

1 small onion, chopped finely
¼pt (150ml) chicken stock
1 large can (14oz/397g) chopped tomatoes
2 cloves garlic, crushed (optional)
Salt and black pepper
Pinch of marjoram
1 tbsp tomato purée
1 tsp cornflour

1. Place the onion in a bowl with 3 tablespoons of stock. Cook on High for 2 minutes.
2. Add the remaining ingredients, except the tomato purée and cornflour.
3. Stir well, cover with perforated cling film, and cook for 5 minutes on High.
4. Remove the cling film, add the tomato purée to the sauce, and the cornflour mixed with a little water. Stir well.
5. Continue cooking for another 5 minutes, stirring once every minute.
6. If you like a smoother sauce, you can whizz it through the food blender before serving.

SCAMPI WITH WHITE WINE AND TOMATO SAUCE

Serves: 4
Calories per serving: 220

This has to be the quickest-ever dinner party dish. If scampi are too expensive, the sauce is equally scrumptious with any firm white fish.

1½lb (750g) frozen uncooked scampi, defrosted
1 small glass dry white wine
1 large onion, chopped finely
2 cloves garlic, crushed
½ small red pepper, cored, deseeded and cubed
3 tomatoes, skinned and chopped
2 tbsp tomato purée
2 tbsp chopped fresh basil or parsley
Salt and black pepper

1.   Place the scampi on a shallow dish, keeping the pieces separate. Pour over the white wine. Cook on High for 2 minutes, stirring after 1 minute.
2.   Transfer the scampi to another dish. Put the onion, garlic and red pepper into the dish containing the wine, and cook on High for 5 minutes.
3.   Add the tomatoes, tomato purée and most of the basil or parsley. Cover with cling film, pierce and cook on High for 5 minutes, stirring once. Season to taste.
4.   Add the scampi, cover and cook on High for 3 minutes. Garnish with the remaining basil or parsley.

COD STEAK ORIENTAL

Serves: 1
Calories per portion: 210

This is scrumptious enough for a dinner party, served with bean sprouts, fluffy rice and salad. Yet, it can be whizzed up in only 4 minutes. You can use the sauce with any white fish, or even with a chicken breast.

8oz (225g) cod fillet, defrosted
1 tsp lemon juice
1 tsp soy sauce
1 tsp tomato juice
Pinch of ground ginger
Salt to taste
1 small orange to garnish
Watercress to garnish

1. Place the cod on a plate or serving dish.
2. Combine the lemon juice, soy sauce, tomato juice and a pinch of ground ginger. Add a little salt to taste.
3. Pour over the fish.
4. Cover and cook on High for 3 minutes or until the fish is cooked.
5. Slice the orange.
6. Remove the fish from the oven, allow to stand, then garnish with orange slices and watercress.

TUNA-STUFFED TOMATOES

Serves: 1
Calories per serving: 150

I love cooking stuffed tomatoes in a micro. It takes just minutes to dish up something that's really tasty and special. In this recipe, I've used tuna as stuffing, but you could also use chopped leftover chicken with brown rice and onion, or wholemeal breadcrumbs with herbs, garlic and a little stock. Serve with plenty of 'free' salad vegetables (see page 35).

One of my other favourite low-calorie tomato tricks is to micro leftover tomato salad (seasoned with lemon juice, wine vinegar and herbs), and throw it on top of a couple of slices of toast. With lashings of Worcestershire sauce and a dollop of cottage cheese, this is a gorgeous breakfast or lunchtime treat for less than 250 calories.

2 large tomatoes
1 small can (3½oz/99g) tuna in brine, drained and
    mashed
½oz (15g) onion, chopped finely
Pinch each of celery salt and dried or chopped fresh
    parsley

1.   Slice the tops off the tomatoes, scoop out the pulp and mix with the remaining ingredients.
2.   Fill the tomatoes, replace the tops and cook on High for 3 minutes.

BAKED POTATO WITH CHEESE AND PRAWNS

Serves: 1
Calories per serving: 275

This is a luxury version of one of our favourite Fatfield lunches. Add masses of salad and vegetables from your 'free' list for a great meal (see page 35). Even if you throw in a glass of dry wine, the calorie total is still under 400, less than a boring old cheese sandwich!

1 8oz (225g) potato, washed, dried and pricked
1oz (25g) red pepper, chopped
2oz (50g) cottage cheese with chives and onion
1½oz (40g) peeled prawns
Chopped parsley to garnish

1.   Place the potato on kitchen paper and cover with another piece of paper.
2.   Microwave on High for 4 minutes.
3.   Turn over and cook for a further 4 minutes. Check that it is cooked through. Leave to stand while preparing the filling.
4.   Mix the pepper with the cottage cheese and prawns.
5.   Split the top of the potato and pile on the filling.
6.   Garnish with chopped parsley and serve with 'free' vegetables.

SUMMER PUDDING

Serves: 6
Calories per serving: 95

You can use fresh or frozen fruit for this traditional recipe, which is actually delicious at any time of the year. Serve it with natural, low-fat yogurt or unsweetened fromage frais.

1½lb (750g) mixed summer fruits (raspberries, blackcurrants, blackberries, redcurrants, cherries, strawberries), fresh or frozen
4fl oz (100ml) unsweetened apple juice
Hermesetas Sprinkle Sweet to taste
5oz (150g) sliced white bread, crusts removed

1. If fresh fruit is used, place in a large bowl with the apple juice. Cover and microwave on High for 4–6 minutes or until lightly cooked, stirring halfway through the cooking time.
2. If using frozen fruit, place it in a large bowl, cover and microwave on Defrost for 8–9 minutes, stirring halfway through the cooking time. Microwave on High for 2 minutes. Stir in the apple juice.
3. Leave the fruit to cool and then add Sprinkle Sweet to taste.
4. Line a 1½pt (850ml) pudding basin with some of the bread.
5. Fill with half of the fruit. Cover with a slice of bread, then top with the remaining fruit.
6. Completely cover the top with the rest of the bread.
7. Place a saucer on top, and weight down with a can of food.
9. Chill for 8 hours or overnight.
9. Turn out the pudding onto a plate to serve.

BAKED APPLE WITH RUM

Serves: 1
Calories per serving: 110

This is just about the lowest-calorie hot dessert you can serve, and it is absolutely delicious. You could add cider or calvados instead of the rum without adding too many extra calories. My assistant, Toni, adds $^{1}/_{2}oz$ (15g) sultanas and a dribble of honey which increases the calorie count to 130. You can add rice pud or semolina for the children.

1 medium cooking apple, cored
1 tbsp rum

1.   Slit the skin around the middle of the apple, and place it in a serving dish. Pour over the liquid.
2.   Cook on High for 2–3 minutes, or until cooked but not mushy.

CHAPTER SEVENTEEN

VEGGIE SLIMSATIONS

If you're green, it's easy to be lean! Not strictly true, I'm afraid, as many vegetarians find that they put on weight once they give up meat. Reasons? It's so tempting to fill up that space on your plate with calorie-loaded foods like cheese, quiches, nuts and creamy pasta dishes. Even vegans, who give up all animal products, sometimes get hooked on high-calorie nibbles and snacks.

But, if you are careful with calories, a veggie diet can be a Fatfield diet, too. Many vegetables can be eaten freely on the diet (check out the list on page 35), so all you have to do is prepare them imaginatively.

Invest in some large, flattish casseroles for cooking superb meals in the oven. Make up tasty vegetable sauces to go with pasta (which contains just 30 calories per 1oz/25g), cooked weight, until you pile cheese and cream on top!) and keep a look out for unusual vegetables like salsify, celeriac, and seakale.

Pulses, such as haricot beans, kidney beans and chick peas, should be kept in every vegetarian store cupboard. Another useful ingredient is Quorn, which is a new food, harvested from a tiny, mushroom-like plant. It is high in fibre and protein, contains no fat or cholesterol and is relatively low in calories.

These recipes will appeal to vegetarians and non-vegetarians alike, but they are not all suitable for vegans.

CHEESE AND VEGETABLE STIR-FRY

Serves: 4
Calories per serving: 160

1lb (450g) mixed crisp vegetables such as carrots, leeks,
    courgettes, sweet peppers, green beans, cauliflower
    and broccoli
1 tbsp sunflower oil
½ tsp each ground cumin, coriander and garam masala
Finely grated rind and juice of 1 large orange
4oz (100g) Edam cheese, cut into ½in (1cm) cubes
4 spring onions, cut into curls to garnish

1.   Wash and dry the vegetables and cut into pieces –
slice leeks, courgettes, carrots and peppers and break
cauliflower and broccoli into florets.
2.   Heat the oil in a heavy-based, non-stick pan over a
medium heat. Add the vegetables and spices and stir-fry
for 2 minutes.
3.   Add the orange rind and juice, bring to the boil, then
reduce the heat and simmer for 3–4 minutes until the
vegetables are just tender.
4.   Add the cheese cubes and stir for a few seconds until
heated through, and the cheese is beginning to melt.
5.   Serve immediately, garnished with spring onion curls.

FRUITY QUORN CURRY

Serves: 3
Calories per serving: 150

Add 4 tablespoons plain, boiled rice and a cool, delicious salad of cucumber with natural, low-fat yogurt and chopped fresh mint, and you'll still consume less than 250 calories! So, who needs a greasy takeaway?

1 tbsp mild curry paste
2 tbsp apricot chutney
1 small can (8oz/227g) chopped tomatoes
1 tbsp sultanas
3 tbsp water
4½ oz (125g) Quorn pieces
1 medium onion, sliced
1 small yellow pepper, cored, deseeded and sliced
1 medium carrot, cut into julienne strips
2oz (50g) mushrooms, sliced
1 stick celery, chopped
1 medium red apple, cored and roughly chopped

1. Mix the curry paste, chutney, tomatoes, sultanas and water in a large pan. Cook, stirring, for 2 minutes.
2. Add the Quorn and onion, cover and simmer for 5 minutes to allow the Quorn to absorb the flavour of the sauce.
3. Add the pepper and carrot and cook for 5 minutes.
4. Add the mushrooms and cook for 1 minute.
5. Add the celery and red apple and heat through.

STUFFED MARROW WITH TOMATO SAUCE

Serves: 4
Calories per serving: 200

1 medium marrow
1oz (25g) grated nuts
4oz (100g) wholemeal breadcrumbs
¼pt (150ml) skimmed milk
Mixed herbs and salt to taste
1 egg
1 small onion, chopped finely
1oz (25g) low-fat spread
½ tsp yeast extract
1oz (25g) low-fat Cheddar cheese, grated
Sauce
1 large can (14oz/397g) chopped tomatoes
1 small onion, chopped finely
1 clove garlic, chopped finely (optional)
1 tsp dried thyme

1.   Wash and scrub the marrow, and cut in half length-wise.
2.   Scoop out the seeds and pith and discard.
3.   Mix together the nuts, breadcrumbs, milk, herbs, salt and egg in a small bowl.
4.   Soften the chopped onion in a little low-fat spread in a saucepan.
5.   Add the stuffing mixture and yeast extract and cook for another minute.
6.   In a large pan, boil the marrow halves for about 5 minutes. Drain.
7.   Place the marrow halves in an ovenproof dish, fill with the stuffing mixture and top with the grated cheese and remaining low-fat spread.

8.   Bake in a moderate oven (325°F, 170°C, gas mark 3) for about 30 minutes or until the marrow is tender. Test with the tip of a pointed knife.
9.   While the marrow is cooking, mix the sauce ingredients in a small saucepan, cover and cook gently for about 20 minutes.
10.   To serve cut each marrow piece in half and pour the sauce on top.

LEEK PIE

Serves: 4
Calories per serving: 160

1lb (450g) leeks, trimmed, washed thoroughly and cut
    into ½in (1cm) slices
1 small carton (5oz/150g) Shape Low Fat Soft Cheese
1lb (450g) potatoes (peeled weight), cooked and mashed
    with ¼pt (150ml) skimmed milk

1.   Boil the leeks in water until cooked but still crisp. Drain thoroughly.
2.   Place the leeks in a shallow, ovenproof dish and mix in the Shape Soft Cheese.
3.   Pile the mashed potato on top, covering the leeks and cheese. Use a fork to decorate the top.
4.   Bake in a moderate oven (375°F, 190°C, gas mark 5) for 25–30 minutes. Flash under the grill just before serving to brown the top.

MIXED VEGETABLE CASSEROLE

Serves: 4
Calories per serving: 60

Non-veggies can serve this delicious casserole with a roast chicken leg, no skin, and still have 'change' out of 350 calories. It is also a super lunch dish, with crusty bread for dunking!

1 tsp low-fat spread
8oz (225g) swede, sliced
2 carrots, sliced
1 large onion, sliced
2 sticks celery, chopped
2 medium leeks, sliced
Salt and black pepper
Pinch of nutmeg
1 large can (14oz/397g) tomatoes
2 tbsp natural, low-fat yogurt
Chopped parsley to garnish

1.   Lightly grease a 3 pint (1.8 litre) casserole with the low-fat spread.
2.   Arrange the vegetables in the dish in layers, sprinkling each layer with seasoning and a pinch of nutmeg.
3.   Pour the tomatoes over the vegetables, cover and cook in a moderate oven (350°F, 180°C, gas mark 4) for about 1 hour, or until the vegetables are tender.
4.   Just before serving, remove the lid, swirl yogurt on top of the tomatoes and sprinkle with chopped parsley.

BRAISED RED CABBAGE WITH APPLE CHEESE

Serves: 2
Calories per serving: 110

This is a favourite dish of successful Fatfield slimmer Linda Philpott, who says it is scrumptious for lunch with a small baked potato and lots of green salad.

1lb (450g) red cabbage, shredded
4oz (100g) cooking apple, cored, peeled and sliced
4oz (100g) onion, sliced
1oz (25g) brown sugar
2 tbsp wine vinegar
4 tbsp water
2oz (50g) Shape Low Fat Soft Cheese
1 cooking apple, cooked and puréed
Salt and black pepper

1. Place the cabbage, apple slices, onion, sugar, vinegar and water in a saucepan. Cover and simmer for 20–30 minutes, until the cabbage is nearly soft.
2. Blend the soft cheese and the apple purée together and stir into the cabbage. Season to taste.

COURGETTES WITH HARICOT BEANS

Serves: 4
Calories per serving: 170

Add 3 tablespoons plain boiled rice, and a leafy green salad for a substantial supper dish that's under 290 calories. Yummy!

6oz (175g) haricot beans, soaked in water overnight
1 large can (14oz/397g) chopped tomatoes
1 green pepper, cored, deseeded and sliced
1 onion, sliced
1 clove garlic, crushed
1lb (450g) courgettes, sliced thickly
2 tsp dried basil
1 small carton (5oz/150g) natural, low-fat yogurt

1.   Drain the beans, cover with fresh water and boil for about 45 minutes, or until tender.
2.   Pour the tomatoes into a large saucepan, add the green pepper, onion, garlic, courgettes and basil, cover and simmer for about 15 minutes, until the vegetables are almost cooked.
3.   Stir in the drained beans, heat through, transfer to a serving dish, and pour the yogurt on top.

FATFIELD PAN HAGERTY

Serves: 4
Calories per serving: 280

The traditional Geordie dish, Pan Hagerty, is usually cooked in a frying pan with lashings of fat. But this version, developed by the Fatfield villagers, is just as delicious, and very filling.

1 tsp low-fat spread
2lb (900g) potatoes (peeled weight), cut into thin slices
1lb (450g) onions, sliced
3oz (75g) low-fat Cheddar cheese, grated
1 carton (5oz/150g) natural, low-fat yogurt
Salt and black pepper

1.   Grease a large, shallow ovenproof dish with the low-fat spread.
2.   Place layers of the potatoes, onions, and grated cheese in the dish, ending with a layer of cheese.
3.   Pour the yogurt evenly over the top, cover loosely with foil and place in a moderate oven (350°F, 180°C, gas mark 4) for 1 hour or until the vegetables are tender.
4.   Remove the foil, and brown the top of the dish under a high grill for a few moments until golden.

SWEET AND SOUR TOFU

Serves: 4
Calories per serving: 385

4oz (100g) long grain brown rice
1lb (450g) tofu, cut into small cubes
1 small bunch spring onions, chopped finely
1 dsp corn oil
1 large can (14oz/397g) tomatoes
1 medium can (15oz/425g) pineapple chunks, canned in
    juice
2oz (50g) whole almonds
4 tbsp soy sauce

1.   Cook the brown rice in plenty of boiling water until still 'nutty' but tender.
2.   In a heavy-based, non-stick pan, fry the tofu and spring onions in the oil very gently for about 3 minutes.
3.   Add the tomatoes, drained pineapple, almonds and soy sauce.
4.   Simmer gently for 5 minutes.
5.   Serve poured over the cooked rice.

ONIONS STUFFED WITH BAKED BEANS

Serves: 2
Calories per serving: 250

4 large onions
1 medium can (7.9oz/225g) curried beans with sultanas
2 tbsp mango chutney, chopped
1 large tomato, chopped
1 tsp low-fat spread for greasing dish (make it less, if
    you can!)
2 tbsp water

1.   Put the peeled onions in a large pan and cover with
cold water. Bring to the boil, cover and simmer for about
35 minutes, or until tender but still firm. Test with the tip
of a pointed knife.
2.   Drain, leave to cool, then cut a small slice from the
base of each onion so it stands firmly.
3.   Remove the centre of each onion with a small spoon,
chop finely and place in a bowl.
4.   Mix the chopped onion with the beans, chutney and
chopped tomato.
5.   Stand the onions in a greased ovenproof dish, pile the
bean stuffing back into the onions, and add the water to the
dish.
6.   Cover and cook for 25 minutes in a hot oven (400°F,
200°C, gas mark 6).

COURGETTES AU GRATIN

Serves: 4
Calories per serving: 230

You can use broccoli, shredded cabbage or leeks instead of courgettes for this dish. Serve it with crusty bread and a crisp green salad.

1 large onion, sliced into rings
1 large can (14oz/397g) chopped tomatoes
2lb (900g) courgettes, sliced into ½in (1cm) pieces
Salt and black pepper
1 tsp dried oregano
8oz (225g) Edam cheese, grated
Chopped parsley to garnish

1.   Place the onion rings and tomatoes in a large, shallow, non-stick saucepan.
2.   Cook gently over a medium heat until the onion is softened.
3.   Add the courgettes, cover and continue cooking for 10 minutes, turning the vegetables to prevent sticking.
4.   Season with salt, freshly ground black pepper and oregano. Stir thoroughly.
5.   Place in a shallow, ovenproof dish and sprinkle with the cheese.
6.   Bake in a moderate oven (375°F, 190°C, gas mark 5) for 20 minutes. Serve sprinkled with chopped parsley.

LENTIL KEDGEREE

Serves: 4–6
Calories per serving: 435 or 300

This can either be served alone as a substantial supper dish for 4 people, or with grilled vegeburgers, in which case there is enough for 6.

12oz (350g) whole brown lentils, soaked and drained
6oz (175g) brown long grain rice
2 tsp curry powder
1 tbsp chopped parsley
Salt and black pepper
1 small onion, sliced thinly
1 red pepper, cored, deseeded and sliced thinly
1 hard-boiled egg, quartered

1.   Cook the lentils in boiling, unsalted water for about 25 minutes, or until tender. Drain.
2.   Meanwhile, cook the rice in boiling, salted water for 30 minutes, or until tender but still 'nutty'. Drain and stir in the curry powder.
3.   Mix together the cooked lentils and rice, stir in most of the parsley, and season to taste.
4.   Pour the mixture into a heated serving dish, and garnish with onion and pepper rings, hard-boiled egg quarters and the rest of the parsley.

BANANA AND NUT SALAD

Serves: 4
Calories per serving: 335

4 medium bananas, sliced
1 large red apple, cored and chopped
2 tbsp lemon juice
4oz (100g) long grain brown rice (dry weight), cooked
    and allowed to cool
4oz (100g) seedless green grapes, halved
2oz (50g) sultanas
2oz (50g) flaked almonds
1oz (25g) chopped walnuts
Lettuce and watercress
1 medium kiwi fruit, sliced

1.   In a large bowl, toss the banana slices and apple in the
lemon juice.
2.   Add the rice, grapes, sultanas, almonds and walnuts
and mix well.
3.   Line a serving dish with lettuce and watercress, place
the banana and nut salad in the centre, and decorate with
slices of kiwi fruit.

PASTA AND WALNUT SALAD

Serves: 4
Calories per serving: 190

Beware of eating too many nuts if you want to slim success-fully. It's best to reserve them for salads such as this deli-cious recipe which is ideal for either lunch or supper.

4oz (100g) wholemeal pasta shapes
3 apples
1 tbsp lemon juice
4 sticks celery, sliced thinly
2 tbsp raisins
1oz (25g) stoned dates, chopped
2 tbsp walnuts, chopped
2 tbsp low-fat, natural yogurt
1 tbsp unsweetened orange juice
Salt and black pepper

1.   Cook the pasta in plenty of boiling, salted water for about 12 minutes, or until just tender. Rinse under a cold tap and drain thoroughly.
2.   Core and thinly slice the apples and toss them in the lemon juice. Stir in the celery, raisins, dates and walnuts.
3.   Fold the fruit and nut mixture into the cooked pasta.
4.   Mix together the yogurt and orange juice, season to taste and pour over the salad, tossing lightly to blend.

CHAPTER EIGHTEEN

WICKED DESSERTS

Are you a pudding-shaped person who loves eating puddings? You don't have to give up delicious desserts just because you want to lose weight. On the Fatfield Diet, you can tuck into scrumptious trifles, marvellous meringues, and tasty tarts and still shed pounds, or even stones! But, I do insist that you follow the diet to the letter. That means that you must eat regularly, and enjoy the main course before you have your dessert. This is to ensure that you are not tempted to 'overdose' on that sweet treat.

The recipes below have all been tried out by our Fatfield villagers who vote them tops for taste and easy preparation. Basic ingredients which are useful for slimmers include sugar-free jams, Hermesetas Sprinkle Sweet (which contains one tenth of the calories of sugar), aerosol cream (one 'squirt' of Anchor aerosol cream is about 10 calories, compared with 55 calories for 1 level tablespoon of double cream), Shape Single (15 calories per 1 level tablespoon), and meringue nests which are just 55 calories each and can be topped with fresh or canned (in juice) fruit to make an instant pud.

Following the Fatfield principle of eating more to weigh less, do make these desserts look even bigger on the plate by adding low-calorie extras. Try slices of melon, grapes, orange slices, or a posh-looking 'coulis', simply a runny fruit purée which is easy to make but looks stunning surrounding a simple pud like slices of mango, peach and pineapple or good old semolina.

LYCHEE AND SHERRY TRIFLE

Serves: 6
Calories per serving: 245

4 trifle sponges
1 tbsp sugar-free jam
4 tbsp sweet sherry
12oz (350g) lychees, fresh or canned in juice
3 egg yolks
2 tsp cornflour
¾pt (425ml) semi-skimmed milk
2 tbsp Hermesetas Sprinkle Sweet
¼pt (150ml) Shape Double
1 kiwi fruit, sliced

1.   Split the trifle sponges and fill with the jam. Place in a glass bowl and dribble over the sherry.
2.   Peel the lychees if using fresh ones or drain canned lychees well and arrange in between and around the sponges.
3.   In a small bowl mix a little milk with the egg yolks and cornflour. Heat the remaining milk until steaming. Pour on to the egg yolks, stirring, and then turn into a small heavy-based, non-stick saucepan.
4.   Cook over a very low heat, stirring all the time, until the custard coats the back of a spoon.
5.   Turn the custard into a basin and stir in the Sprinkle Sweet. Pour the custard over the lychees and sponges and leave until cold.
6.   Whip the Shape Double and pipe or spread on the trifle.
7.   Decorate with slices of kiwi fruit.

RASPBERRY PAVLOVA

Serves: 6
Calories per serving: 240

This is a treat from down under, that will help you slim your down under, too! It consists of a basic meringue base, topped with Shape Double and fresh or frozen raspberries. You can, of course, use other fruit such as strawberries or mandarin oranges.

3 egg whites
6oz (175g) caster sugar
1 tsp cornflour
½ tsp vanilla essence
½ tsp white vinegar
½pt (275ml) Shape Double
8oz (225g) fresh or frozen raspberries

1.   Preheat the oven to 300°F, 150°C, gas mark 2. Draw a 7in (18cm) circle on a piece of non-stick baking paper. Place on a baking sheet.
2.   Whisk the egg whites until very stiff. Mix the sugar with the cornflour and whisk in 1 tablespoon at a time, beating until stiff after each addition. Whisk in the vanilla essence and vinegar.
3.   Spoon or pipe the mixture on to the paper to cover the circle. Reduce the oven to 275°F, 140°C, gas mark 1 and bake for 50–60 minutes or until crisp on top but still soft in the middle. Leave to cool and then peel off the paper.
4.   Whip the Shape Double until it holds its shape. Place the meringue base on a plate and spoon the Double on top.
5.   Decorate with raspberries.

APRICOT AND YOGURT ICECREAM

Serves: 6
Calories per serving: 105

This is so quick to make that you'll wonder why you never thought of making your own icecream before. The saving in calories and fat is considerable. You can adapt the recipe to use with other fruit canned in juice, such as pineapple, mandarin oranges or cherries.

1 large can (15oz/425g) apricots in natural juice
1pt (575ml) natural, whole milk yogurt
Almond essence to taste

1.   Drain the apricots, reserving the juice.
2.   Liquidize or mash the fruit to a pulp.
3.   In a large bowl, mix together the apricot purée and yogurt. Add 3 tablespoons of the apricot juice and almond essence to taste.
4.   Turn the mixture into a freezer container. Cover and freeze until almost solid. Then whisk or beat in a food processor to break down the ice crystals.
5.   Return the icecream to the freezer and freeze until solid.
6.   Remove the icecream from the freezer 30 minutes before serving and place in the fridge to soften slightly.

STRAWBERRY OR MANDARIN CHOCOLATE ROLL

Serves: 8
Calories per serving: 115

This is the best-ever pud for reformed chocoholics. It contains cocoa to give you a lift, but the fromage frais provides protein to help stop you from craving another slice! Strawberries are great for this when available, but it is equally delicious with mandarins, canned in juice.

3 large eggs (size 2), separated
4 tbsp Hermesetas Sprinkle Sweet
1½oz (40g) self-raising flour
1oz (25g) drinking chocolate powder
3 tbsp hot water
4 tbsp low-sugar strawberry jam
8oz (225g) fromage frais
4oz (100g) strawberries or mandarins, canned in juice

1.   Grease and line a 12 × 9in (30 × 23cm) Swiss roll tin with non-stick baking parchment.
2.   Whisk the egg yolks with the Sprinkle Sweet until light and creamy.
3.   Sieve together the flour and the drinking chocolate and fold into the yolk mixture with the hot water.
4.   Whisk the egg whites until stiff but not dry and fold gently into the egg yolks. Turn the mixture into the prepared tin and bake in a hot oven (400°F, 200°C, gas mark 6) for 12–15 minutes or until the sponge springs back when lightly pressed.
5.   Turn out onto a large sheet of greaseproof paper. Quickly trim off the edges and peel off the lining paper. Then roll up with the greaseproof paper inside. Leave to cool.

6. Unroll the sponge gently and spread with the jam, then the fromage frais.
7. Reserve some of the fruit for decoration, and slice the rest. Place the sliced fruit on top of the fromage frais.
8. Re-roll the sponge and place carefully on a serving dish.
9. Decorate with the reserved fruit and a little Sprinkle Sweet.

TONI'S LOW-CALORIE SEMOLINA

Serves: 2–3
Calories per serving: For 2, 90; for 3, 60

Fatfield slimming counsellor, Toni Tompsett, whizzes up this basic semolina to feed her family – and herself. She adds a teaspoon of low-calorie jam (adds 10 calories), a pinch of ground nutmeg, or fruit. Occasionally, she mixes it with natural, low-fat yogurt.

½pt (275ml) skimmed milk
¾oz (20g) semolina
Hermesetas Sprinkle Sweet to taste

1. Heat the milk in a small pan nearly to boiling point.
2. Stir in the semolina, and cook gently for 2 minutes, stirring all the time.
3. Remove from the heat and stir in the sweetener before serving.

COLD RHUBARB CRUMBLE

Serves: 4
Calories per serving: 90

Everyone has a favourite crumble recipe, but for slimmers the main problem is that most crumbles need butter in the topping. This one is different because the topping is simply crushed digestive biscuits. The rhubarb is absolutely delicious mixed with a carton of low-fat rhubarb yogurt. Use the same recipe with apple purée mixed with low-fat blackcurrant yogurt, or raspberries with raspberry or mandarin low-fat yogurt.

1lb (450g) rhubarb, chopped
Grated rind and juice of 1 orange
A little Hermesetas Sprinkle Sweet to taste
1 carton (4½oz/125g) low-fat rhubarb yogurt
4 medium digestive biscuits, crushed
½ tsp mixed spice
Orange slices to decorate

1.   Put the rhubarb, orange rind and juice in a large pan. Stew until soft, then leave to cool.
2.   Blend the mixture in a blender or pass through a sieve to make a purée. Add the sweetener to taste.
3.   Stir in the yogurt, and pour into 1 large, or 4 individual glass bowls.
4.   Mix the biscuits with the mixed spice and spoon over the fruit. Chill.
5.   Decorate with orange slices, and serve.

LINDISFARNE CREAM

Serves: 6
Calories per serving: 140

This is a traditional Geordie dish, using the wonderful mead which comes from the island of Lindisfarne. In this recipe, it is made the low-calorie way. If you don't like mead, you can use sweet sherry instead. Children may prefer it made with apple or orange juice.

1lb (450g) cooking apples, peeled, cored and sliced
3 eggs, separated
2 tbsp Hermesetas Sprinkle Sweet
2 tsp powdered gelatine
3 tbsp water
1 tbsp lemon juice
1 tbsp mead, preferably from Lindisfarne
¼pt (150ml) Shape Double to decorate

1. Cook the apples in a little water until soft. Mash well or purée and allow to cool.
2. In a large bowl whisk together the egg yolks and Sprinkle Sweet until pale and creamy.
3. Fold in the apple purée.
4. Prepare the gelatine by sprinkling it onto 3 tablespoons of cold water in a cup. Leave to stand for 5 minutes. Place the cup in a pan containing a little simmering water and leave until the gelatine is dissolved. Or microwave on Defrost for 30 seconds. Stir the dissolved gelatine into the apple mixture, together with the lemon juice and mead.
5. Beat the egg whites until stiff and fold into the mixture.
6. Pour into a glass dish, and chill until set.
7. Decorate with whipped Shape Double.

SLIMMERS' APPLE BREAD PUDDING

Serves: 4
Calories per serving: 215

This pud is full of fibre, and so filling that you probably won't be able to get up from the table without groaning. Children will love this, served hot for supper, with a scoop of home-made icecream on top.

4 large slices wholemeal bread
1oz (25g) sultanas
³⁄₄pt (425ml) semi-skimmed milk
2 eggs
Vanilla essence to taste
3 apples, cored and thinly sliced
¼ tsp ground nutmeg
¼ tsp ground cinnamon

1.   Cut the bread slices into quarters and line a shallow ovenproof dish. Sprinkle with the sultanas.
2.   Lightly beat the milk and eggs in a bowl, add a few drops of vanilla essence, and strain over the bread. Leave to stand for 30 minutes.
3.   Top with the apple slices, and sprinkle with nutmeg and cinnamon.
4.   Bake for 30–40 minutes in a moderate oven (350°F, 180°C, gas mark 4) until set. Flash under a hot grill to make the apples go golden brown.

CHOCOLATE MOUSSE

Serves: 4
Calories per serving: 80

Everyone's favourite pud, but strictly out of bounds for slimmers? Not if you make it this way, discovered by Toni!

1 carton (7.7oz/215g) Carnation Light unsweetened
    condensed semi-skimmed milk
2 tsp powdered gelatine
4 tbsp water
1 sachet Ovaltine Options Choc-Orange or Choc-o-Lait
    drink
Mandarin segments to decorate

1.   Chill the carton of Carnation Light overnight in the fridge.
2.   Sprinkle the gelatine onto 2 tablespoons of cold water in a cup. Leave to soak for 5 minutes. Stand the cup in a pan containing a little simmering water and leave until the gelatine is dissolved. Or microwave on Defrost for 30 seconds.
3.   Mix the Ovaltine Options with 2 tablespoons hot water to a smooth paste.
4.   Whip the Carnation Light until very frothy. Continue whipping and adding the dissolved gelatine and chocolate mixture.
5.   Turn into a serving dish or 4 individual dishes and chill until set. Decorate with mandarin segments.

SIX QUICK AND EASY PUDS

Serves: 1

1.   Bake 1 large banana with the juice of ½ orange and a pinch of cinnamon. *Calories: 125.*

2.   Place one 5oz (150g) pot of Ambrosia Light Rice on a dish, top with ½ a peach, canned in juice. Sprinkle with cinnamon and flash under the grill. *Calories: 130.*

3.   Place 1 small ready-made meringue nest on a plate, top with a few green grapes and 1 tablespoon low-fat fromage frais. *Calories: 90.*

4.   Make a crunchy 'sundae' with layers of low fat fruit yogurt, chopped fresh fruit and bran flakes. Calories using 1 carton (4½oz/125g) Diet Ski yogurt, 1 pear, ½oz (15g) Bran Flakes: *150.*

5.   Put 2oz (50g) blackberries in a dish, slosh on 1 tablespoon cassis liqueur and top with 1 tablespoon natural, low-fat yogurt. *Calories: 70.*

6.   Make your own mini 'cheesecake' by crumbling 1 digestive biscuit in a dish and adding 1 tablespoon low-fat soft cheese and a squeeze of lemon juice. *Calories: 100,* or, double everything up for just *200* calories!

FATFIELD FAVOURITES

Here's a list of branded foods and drinks which our Fatfield slimmers found especially helpful and delicious on the diet:

FOOD	SIZE	CALORIES
Breakfast Cereals		
Kellogg's Sultana Bran	1oz (25g)	91
Quaker Puffed Wheat	1oz (25g)	93
Shredded Wheat	1	80
Weetabix	1	65
Cereal Bars		
Quaker Harvest Crunch		
Chocolate and Raisin	1	80
Crispbreads		
Ryvita Original	1 slice	25
RyKing Brown	1 slice	35
Dairy Products		
St Ivel Shape Soft Cheese with		
Garlic and Herbs	150g pot	200
Shape Full Flavoured Cheddar		
Type	1oz (25g)	73
Shape Fromage Frais	100g pot	
Apricot or orange flavour		60
Strawberry or raspberry		
flavour		65
Shape French Style Set		
Yogurts	125g pot	50
St Ivel Gold	1oz (25g)	110
Diet Ski Yogurts	125g pot	50
Delight Half Fat Cheddar cheese	1oz (25g)	80

Delight Half Fat Cheese Spread Portions	1	35
Low Fat Dairy Spread with Medium Fat Cheese	1oz (25g)	52
Low Fat Soft Cheese with Garlic and Herbs	1oz (25g)	42
Delight Extra Low	1oz (25g)	56

Drinks

Ovaltine Options, all flavours	1 cup	40
Boots Shapers Apple and Blackberry drink (undiluted)	1fl oz (28ml)	2
McEwans LA low-alcohol beer	440ml can	65
John Smith's low alcohol bitter	½pt/275ml bottle	45
Eisberg Alcohol Free Wine	1 glass	35

Puddings

Bird's Sugar Free Jelly	1 pack	45
Ambrosia Devon Custard	150g pot	150
Ross Mousse, all flavours	1 tub	90

Ready Meals

Findus Lean Cuisine:

Chili Con Carne	1 pack	275
Kashmiri Chicken Curry	1 pack	275
Cod Mornay	1 pack	180
Spaghetti Bolognaise	1 pack	240
Lamb Tikka Masala	1 pack	260
Chicken à l'Orange with Almond Rice	1 pack	270
Beef and Pork Cannelloni with Mornay Sauce	1 pack	235

FATFIELD FAVOURITES

Batchelors Slim a Meals:

Chicken Risotto, Beef Risotto, Chow Mein, Paella	1 pack	250

Snacks

Golden Wonder Pot Noodles:

Beef and Tomato	1 pot	315
Chicken and Mushroom	1 pot	330
Chow Mein	1 pot	325
Spicy Beef Curry	1 pot	340

Soups

Batchelors Slim a Soups, all flavours	1 sachet	40
Batchelors Slim a Soup Specials, all flavours	1 sachet	60
Heinz Weight Watchers Soups	10.4oz/295g can	
Celery	1 can	60
Chicken	1 can	65
Chicken Noodle or Minestrone	1 can	55

Spreads

Delight Ardennes or Brussels Pâté	1oz (25g)	61
Shippams Salmon or Sardine and Tomato Paste	1.23oz (35g) pot	50

Sweeteners

Hermesetas Sprinkle Sweet	1 tsp	2

WHAT SHOULD YOU WEIGH?

Don't aim too low when you are deciding
on your goal weight. As I have said before, the best weight for
you is the one at which you feel and look good. It may well be
that a certain amount of plumpness suits you!
Below is a chart for recording your weekly weight-loss.
Weigh in on the same scales, at the same time of day. Measure
your chest, waist, and hips at the same time – and don't cheat
by pulling your tape-measure in too tightly.

DATE	WEIGHT	BUST	WAIST	HIPS

YOUR FOOD DIARY

During the first, difficult weeks of your diet, it is a good idea to keep a food diary. Note *exactly* what you ate, and how you felt when you ate it. If you cheated, you must include all the naughty nibbles and drinks which were not on your official Fatfield food plan.

Every week, sit down quietly, and go through the diary. Try to plan a strategy for dealing with difficult moments that crop up again and again. For instance, if you always seem to nibble bread and butter when you are cutting sandwiches for your childrens' tea, make sure you have a mug of slimmer's soup handy to sip instead.

If you habitually go astray when the 11am snack trolley comes round the office, make sure you are *out* of the room at that time or have some fresh fruit in your desk to eat instead of a fattening snack.

Make yourself a diary like this, and keep it daily:

	Breakfast	*Lunch*	*Supper*	*Drinks and Nibbles*
MONDAY				
Place	ON THE BUS	AT WORK	AT HOME	THE PUB
Time	8·30AM	1PM	6PM	9PM
What I ate	BAG OF SWEETS	WHOLEMEAL SANDWICH FRUIT	FATFIELD SHEPHERD'S PIE	GIN & TONIC PORK PIE
How I felt	CROSS WITH MYSELF!	VIRTUOUS!	FULL UP!	A BIT DOWN (SHOULD HAVE EATEN A BETTER BREAKFAST!)

295

Breakfast	Lunch	Supper	Drinks and Nibbles

Breakfast	*Lunch*	*Supper*	*Drinks and Nibbles*

Breakfast	Lunch	Supper	Drinks and Nibbles

	Breakfast	Lunch	Supper	Drinks and Nibbles

*Breakfast   Lunch   Supper   Drinks
                                     and
                                     Nibbles*

Breakfast	*Lunch*	*Supper*	*Drinks and Nibbles*

Breakfast	Lunch	Supper	Drinks and Nibbles

Breakfast	Lunch	Supper	Drinks and Nibbles

SIGN ON AND SLIM DOWN

One of the best ways to motivate yourself to lose weight, is to make a pact with the one person who will be affected most by your success or failure – *you!*

As I explained in Chapter Seven, it is a good idea to sign some kind of pledge which you can keep safely – perhaps pinned on the kitchen wall – until you have lost weight. Or, get someone such as your partner, your doctor (or even *me!*) to keep it safely for you.

We have a special Fatfield Charter (*see* opposite), which we ask our slimmers to fill in before they start our diet. The simple act of writing down your aims will start you off on the correct footing for successful slimming.

If you want to send your completed Charter to me, include details of your weight problems, plus a polaroid photograph. Include your full name and address and daytime telephone number.

When you reach the targets set out in your Charter, send me another Polaroid picture, with details of your achievement. I will return the Charter to you, endorsed with the Fatfield Seal of Excellence!

The address is: Fatfield Charter, Sally Ann Voak, PO Box 618, Coulsdon, Surrey CR5 1RU.

THE FATFIELD CHARTER

I, ... , promise to follow the Fatfield Diet faithfully and diligently until I lose a total of . . . . lb in weight.

I aim to reach that target on . . . . (date)

Forsaking all other diets, I will remain true to the Fatfield principles of eating large, healthy meals.

I will try not to cheat, but if I do fall by the wayside I will not feel guilty. Instead, I will pull myself together and make up for my transgressions on the following day!

I will also endeavour to take more exercise. This is an outline of my exercise plan . . . .
. . . .
. . . .

When I have lost 7lb I promise that I will give myself a present or treat, such as . . . .

When I have lost 1 stone, I promise that I will give myself a more expensive gift or larger treat, such as
. . . .

When I reach my goal weight, I will buy myself something very special indeed, such as . . . .
. . . .

Signed this day . . . . (date),

in the presence of

Witness No. One . . . . (signature)

Witness No. Two . . . . (signature)

INDEX OF RECIPES